The Family and Community Life of Older People

Family life has changed rapidly over the past fifty years, the growth in the proportion of older people in the population providing a major influence. *The Family and Community Life of Older People* revisits three areas (Bethnal Green in London, Wolverhampton in the Midlands and Woodford in Essex) which were the subject of classic studies in the late 1940s and 1950s, and explores changes to the family and community lives of older people. The book examines issues such as:

- changes in household composition
- changes in the geographical proximity of kin and relatives
- the extent and type of help provided by the family
- contact and relationships with neighbours
- relationships with friends
- involvement in social and leisure activities
- experiences of minority ethnic groups.

These questions are explored through a unique set of data including census material and survey data from interviews with over six hundred older people. A key finding is that over the past fifty years we have moved from an old age experienced within the context of the family group to one shaped by personal communities in which friends may feature as significantly as immediate kin and relatives.

The Family and Community Life of Older People is a major contribution to the sociology of the family, of ageing, and of urban life, and addresses the key social policy issues for an ageing society.

Chris Phillipson is Professor of Applied Social Studies and Gerontology, University of Keele, **Miriam** Gerontology and Head of the School of Soci **Judith Phillips** is Senior Lecturer in Social W Keele, **Jim Ogg** is a Research Associate at the Vieillissement, CNAV. Paris.

The Family and Community Life of Older People

Social networks and social support in three urban areas

Chris Phillipson,
Miriam Bernard, Judith Phillips
and Jim Ogg

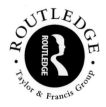

ROUTLEDGE
Taylor & Francis Group

London and New York

First published 2001 by Routledge
11 New Fetter Lane, London EC4P 4EE

Simultaneously published in the USA and Canada
by Routledge
29 West 35th Street, New York, NY 10001

Routledge is an imprint of the Taylor & Francis Group

Typeset in Times and Gill Sans by
Curran Publishing Services Ltd, Norwich
Printed and bound in Great Britain by
Biddles Ltd, Guildford and King's Lynn

British Library Cataloguing in Publication Data
A catalogue record for this book is available
from the British Library

Library of Congress Cataloging in Publication Data
The family and community life of older people: social networks
and social support in three urban areas / by Chris Phillipson
. . . [et al.].
304pp 13.8 x 21.6 cm
Includes bibliographical references and index.
  1. Aged–England–London. 2. Aged–England–Wolverhampton.
  3. Aged–England–Woodford. 4. Aged–Social networks–
England–London. 5. Aged–Social networks–England–
  Wolverhampton. 6. Aged–Social networks–England–
  Woodford. 7. Aged–Services for England–London. 8.Aged–
  Services for–England–Wolverhampton. 9. Aged–Services for–
England–Woodford. 10. Aged–England–London–Family
  relationships. 11. Aged–England–Wolverhampton–Family
  relationships. 12. Aged–England–Woodford–Family
  relationships. 13. Bethnal Green (London, England)
  I. Phillipson, Chris.

  HQ1064.G7 F36 2000
  305.26'0942–dc21   00–32211

ISBN 0–415–20530–1 (hbk)
ISBN 0–415–20531–X (pbk)

To Frank Glendenning:
educationalist and intrepid researcher

Contents

Plates

Tables

Copyright acknowledgements

Acknowledgements

This book is based upon a research study funded by the Economic and Social Research Council (ESRC), as part of their Research Programme on Population and Household Change. The authors gratefully acknowledge the financial support provided by the ESRC. During the life of the project, a range of people and organisations provided help and advice of different kinds. Social and Community Planning Research undertook the survey work for the study with great efficiency and adherence to deadlines. A variety of staff in the social services departments in Wolverhampton and the London Borough of Tower Hamlets assisted with the research at different times. In Wolverhampton, extensive help was provided by Martin Shreeve (Director of Social Services), Anne Bailey, Pat Reader, Kate Read, and members of the Department's team of interpreters (particularly Satwan Sagoo). In Tower Hamlets the research team had excellent support from Emdadul Haque, Saheed Ullah and Mel Wright. Toni Antonucci provided valuable help at an early stage of the research. Peter Willmott, Tony Warnes, and Michael Young gave generously of their time to comment upon different aspects of the research. We are indebted to their wise advice and guidance. Susan McRae, Director of the Population and Household Change Programme, was highly supportive throughout the work. The project team also benefited from advice from researchers on other projects in the Programme. The project received excellent secretarial support and we would like to thank in particular Mary Parker and Sue Allingham. Keele University provided valuable periods of sabbatical leave to the grantholders during the life of the project, and this assisted greatly in the development of the study. We are very grateful indeed to the 627 older people who participated in the research (in all cases, names of these interviewees have been changed to preserve their anonymity). We have also benefited greatly at different stages of the work from the advice of colleagues in the Centre for Social Gerontology at Keele. Final responsibility for the conduct of the research and the presentation of findings rests, of course, with the authors of this book.

Chris Phillipson, Miriam Bernard,
Judith Phillips, Jim Ogg
Keele, August 2000

Part 1

Background to the research

Chapter 1

Growing old

Other pasts; other places

> It was like a country remembering its history: the past was never just the past, it was what made the present able to live with itself.
>
> (Julian Barnes, *England, England*)

Introduction

The aim of this book is to explore changes to the social and family networks of older people living in three urban areas of England: Bethnal Green in London, Wolverhampton in the Midlands and Woodford in Essex. These localities were the subject of different studies in the 1940s and 1950s, many of which examined the changing character of family and community life.[1] Our task has been to return to these areas and to explore the way in which life has altered some fifty years on from those original studies. In this book we pose the question: how different is it to be an older person now in comparison with the 1950s? The treatment of older people is invariably the subject of comparisons with previous times. Indeed, elderly people are often seen to represent the past, conveying a sense of how life has changed from some distant point. But drawing a distinction between the middle and end of the twentieth century has particular resonance. Our sense of the immediate period after the war (conveyed in studies by Peter Willmott, Michael Young and Peter Townsend amongst others) is of older people embedded in complex family ties or what Frankenburg was to describe as an 'environment of kin'.[2] Such ties were seen as central in shaping movement through the life course, from birth through marriage, employment and retirement, to eventual death.

Research in the late 1940s and 1950s examined the thesis that, in the context of a developing welfare state, families were increasingly leaving the old to fend for themselves. The findings from this work, however, suggested a different picture. Most of the studies demonstrated the continuing importance of kinship and family life in post-war Britain. Sheldon, for example, described Wolverhampton society as one in which the old are an essential part of family life. He questioned whether the phrase 'living alone' was in fact of any value in Wolverhampton, given the high degree of residential proximity of kin to elderly people. Townsend also reported on a community that, despite the devastation suffered during the war, appeared to be remarkably successful in its provision of support to older people. Alongside this, however, the studies also stressed the desire of older people to sustain an independent life: a desire which earlier generations of elders would have recognised, and which future generations have maintained.[3]

Similarly, it was the concern of Willmott's and Young's study of Woodford to explore the extent to which geographical and social mobility may have loosened ties between generations. In fact, what they referred to as the 'surprise' of their study was the degree of similarity in many important respects between middle-class Woodford and working-class Bethnal Green. In terms of regular contact and geographical proximity, they were led to the conclusion that 'The old people of the suburb are plainly as much as in touch with children, measured in this way, as those in the East End'.[4] There were, though, some important differences between life in a working-class inner-city community and in a more affluent suburb. One was that, in the former, the generations lived side by side throughout life; in the latter, this tended to follow on from a bereavement. Increasing mobility, while not preventing links between the generations, did tend to loosen traditional obligations. Given this background, and forty to fifty years on from these original investigations, this book set out to explore how the lives of older people had changed in the intervening years.

The earlier research had confirmed that despite the establishment of a welfare state (and partly because of its inadequacies) the family remained of fundamental importance in shaping the lives of older people. As Peter Townsend expressed it: 'To the old person as much as the young it seems to be the supreme comfort and support. Its central purpose is as strong as ever.'[5] This locking together of the old with the family (and in particular the extended family) had both negative and positive consequences. Positively, it confirmed that older people were not just in touch with kin, but that such ties were available to provide different forms of support. More negatively, however, it seemed to fix older people as being in some way inseparable from the family. The sociology of old age became invariably a sociology of the family and not much else. Moreover, given that the family, with greater social mobility, rising female employment, and increased prosperity, was being transformed, older people were seen as disadvantaged by such change. Because the family was doing other things, had other tasks and interests, older people came to be seen as on the periphery rather than at the centre of informal relationships. This view was most clearly expressed in functionalist social theory, which was influential from the 1950s to the late 1960s.[6] But it appeared in other forms as well, for example in the guise of modernisation theory as developed in the 1970s by Cowgill and Holmes.[7] Although the arguments associated with these theories have been challenged in different types of studies, the view that older people are adversely affected by change has been highly influential. It is precisely this perception that is explored in the research discussed in this book.

The experience of modernity

Drawing a comparison between the position of older people at the middle, in contrast with the end, of the twentieth century is significant for reasons other than those already cited. The 1950s were, as Conekin *et al.* suggest, a decisive watershed in Britain's economic and social history.[8] Crook *et al.*, in their analysis of the characteristics of modernity, argue that: 'For a period around the middle of the twentieth century . . . it became possible to elaborate a vision of modernity in which a predictable, progressive and fundamentally benign process of 'modernization' would become diffused throughout the world'.[9]

Reconstructing old age became an important component within this agenda. Growing old was to be moved from its association with the poor law, to a new identity built around social rights attached to citizenship (a theme identified by T. H. Marshall in his essay *Citizenship and Social Class*).[10] Moreover, there was greater awareness that the population was now ageing. The first half of the century had seen a transformation in Britain's demography. In 1901, almost a third of the British population was under the age of fifteen, with just 5 per cent over sixty-five. By 1951, less than a quarter of the population was under fifteen, and more than 10 per cent over sixty-five. But the image of an 'ageing society' hardly captured the mood of the times. If we summarise what it meant to be an older person in, say, the early 1950s, a number of features stand out. As a birth cohort, this is a group born in the mid- to late-nineteenth century: one which had matured with the twentieth century. Their most recent significant historical experience was the Second World War, the impact of which was an important backdrop to our baseline studies. Interviewing older people (Londoners especially) in the late 1940s and early 1950s captured a population trying to shake itself free from disturbing memories of the immediate past; a generation 'made tired by the war' as Doris Lessing expresses it in her memoir of life in the 1950s.[11] And older people in the cities (though less so the 'metro-land' of suburban Woodford) would have been caught up in the dilapidated urban environment: a combination of the 1930s depression and wartime bombing.

The blitz destroyed or damaged 3.5 million homes in metropolitan London. East End boroughs such as Stepney, Poplar and Bethnal Green lost around 19 per cent of their built-up area. But many of the houses which were standing in London, Wolverhampton and other large cities, reflected as much pre-First World War living standards (when in fact the vast majority had been built). Inwood, in his *History of London*, notes that in 1951 18 per cent of households were sharing a bath with another family; one in three shared a lavatory; and 16 per cent a kitchen sink.[12] The Nuffield Committee's report on older people, which surveyed some London boroughs, Wolverhampton and a number of other industrial areas, commented on the lack of bathrooms in the homes of older people:

> Of the houses visited, 28 per cent in Wandsworth and 57 per cent in St Pancras had no bathrooms, and arrangements for preparing and emptying a bath in a flat in a converted house, where the stairs may be steep and taps and sinks few and far between, impose a heavy burden on an older person.[13]

In Wolverhampton, only one in three houses visited had an inside toilet; 6 per cent had already been condemned for slum clearance. The general sense of squalor in urban areas seemed to penetrate all aspects of daily life. Doris Lessing captures this point vividly:

> The London of the late 1940s, the early 1950s, has vanished, and now it is hard to believe it existed. It was unpainted, buildings were stained and cracked and dull and grey; it was war-damaged, some areas all ruins, and under them holes full of dirty water, once cellars, and it was subject to sudden dark fogs – that was before the Clean Air Act. . . . Clothes were still 'austerity' from the war, dismal and ugly. Everyone was indoors by ten, and the streets were

empty. . . . Rationing was still on. The war still lingered, not only in
the bombed places but in people's minds and behaviour. Any conversation tended to drift towards the war, like an animal licking a
sore place. There was wariness, a weariness.[14]

In one sense, this is the 'backward-looking' part of the post-war society
which older people (as survivors) perhaps most clearly represented.
Elderly people clung to their family as a reassuring landmark in a
shifting, more mobile society. As a 'nineteenth century' generation,
though, they had been part of the revolution affecting fertility.[15] In the
second half of the nineteenth century, 43 per cent of the population
would have been brought up in a family with seven or more children; by
1950 this had fallen to just 2 per cent. Studies of older people in the
1950s were in fact on the cusp of a revolution in family life. Those born
at the earliest point of the cohort (all of those in Sheldon's study of
Wolverhampton in 1945 and many of those in the Bethnal Green studies
in the early 1950s) still reflect a pattern where more than two children
was the norm (nearly one in three of Townsend's sample had five or
more surviving children), and where a child staying in the home for part
or all of an older person's old age was also normal. By the end of the
1950s, however, both these aspects had undergone change, with the
consolidation of trends towards smaller family size, as well as a growth
in the proportion of older people living alone.

Yet it is not entirely convincing to see the 1950s as a period defined
by 'extended' families protecting people from misfortune and personal
breakdown. That is one image certainly, powerfully conveyed in studies
of the time. On the other hand, there were also signs of people unable
to connect in certain respects with an urban society that was highly
pressurised (a theme explored in the Chicago school of urban ethnogra-
phy in the 1930s and 1940s).[16] This was especially true for the
newly-arrived migrants from the Caribbean, whose first arrival on the
Empire Windrush in 1948 is now viewed as a turning point in British
social history.[17] Sam Selvon's *The Lonely Londoners*, a moving account
of immigrant life in London in the 1950s, is a reminder of the fragmentation and detachment from the community which could exist alongside
the dense social networks of Bethnal Green.[18] A character in the novel
describes the likely fate for Caribbeans who stayed on in London into
their old age:

Fellers like you would stay in Brit'n till you dead. You come like
old spade I know. He living down Ladbroke Grove. He come to this

country since he was a young man, full of ambition, and he never went back. He had some good times, yes, but what you think happen to him in old age? If you see him now, crouching about in them tube station in a old beast coat, and picking cigarette butt from the pavement. Study for old age, boy. Study what will happen to you if you stay here and get old.[19]

Behind this anxiety is the estrangement of the migrant (and cities such as London and Wolverhampton were certainly in some form or another societies of migrants). Another character in Selvon's book describes his life in the following way:

This [London] is a lonely miserable city, if it was that we didn't get together now and then to talk about tings back home, we would suffer like hell. Here is not like home where you have your friends all about. In the beginning you would think that is a good thing, that nobody minding your business, but after a while you want to get in company, you want to go on excursion to the sea. . . . Nobody in London does really accept you. They tolerate you, yes, but you can't go in their house and eat or sit down and talk. It ain't have no family life for us here.[20]

And there was always the fear of dropping completely through the net and becoming lost in what Ruth Glass (in an early study of West Indian migrants) termed 'the zone of transition'.[21] Interestingly, Selvon illustrates this by evoking what were to become fears expressed in the 1970s and 1980s about the possibility of dying alone without relatives:

And another thing look how people does dead and nobody don't know nothing until the milk bottles start to pile up at the front door. Supposing one day I keel off here in this room? I don't take milk regular – I would stay here until one of the boys drop round. That is a hell of a thing to think about, you know. One time a test dead in this house-right there down the hall, in the second room. You know what? I miss the test – was one of them old geezers, every morning she see me she say. 'Cold today isn't it? I bet you wish you were back home now.' She used to wear a fur coat and go in the park and sit down, crouch up like a fowl when rain falling. Well I miss the test: when I asked the landlord for her, he say she dead about a month ago. You see what I mean?[22]

In contrast, the pessimism of the migrant (reinforced by widespread racial discrimination in the 1950s) was countered by the optimism of those feeling greater prosperity after the restrictions of the early post-year years. Rationing finally ended in 1954, with 'housewives ceremoniously [tearing] up their ration books in Trafalgar Square'.[23] By the mid-1950s, the latest gadgets and home appliances were starting to become affordable: 'Everyone aspired to model their homes on a G Plan "look", the radical textile design, the Dansette record player and, in the kitchen, the food mixer, electric fridge and hygenic formica surfaces'.[24] This was matched by what Gardiner, in her book *From the Bomb to the Beatles*, views as the new 'science' which was to become 'the aesthetic of the 1950s'. Among its elements she lists: the discovery (in 1952) of DNA; the invention of the contraceptive pill (also in 1952); vaccination against polio (1955); the development of the radio telescope (1956); and the exploration of outer space with the launch of the Russian sputniks (1957). This brave new world was described in A. S. Byatt's novel *The Virgin in the Garden* (itself set in the 1950s) as:

> a broad consensus, no class conflict, only within reach, equality of opportunity. A time when most British people believed modestly and without excitement in better things to come as better things had come, bananas, oranges, the Health Service, the Butler Education Act, plans to expand higher education, motor cars for working men.[25]

Women and the absence of men

The place of older people in this new age was unclear, with older men emerging as a group experiencing particular difficulties. An important feature of the 1950s, striking both from the photographic record and the urban sociology of the time, is the apparent marginalisation of the elderly male, most notably in working-class urban areas. An early paperback version of Willmott and Young's *Family and Kinship in East London*, depicts on its front cover a group of four women and two children.[26] At the edge of the scene, uninvolved and ignored by the women, is an elderly man. He seems to be playing the role of court jester to the group, his own dependency matching that of the children. This social redundancy is also brought out in a series of photographs documenting social changes in a Yorkshire mining village from the 1930s onwards.[27] The photographs of the 1950s are especially striking. On the one hand are inter-generational groups of women – from young

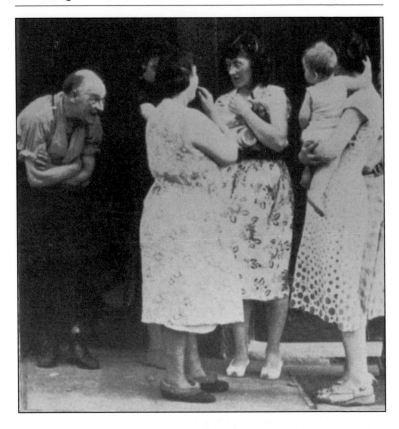

Plate 1: Street scene in London in the early 1950s

Note: This photograph was reproduced on the front cover of early paperback editions of *Family and Kinship in East London*, by Michael Young and Peter Wilmott

children to grandmothers – grouped together in animated conversation. On the other hand, are groups of elderly men, huddled on street corners, expressing a loss of purpose and identity (the comparison with photographs of the unemployed in the 1930s is fairly exact here).

This photographic record (reflecting a tradition of presenting older people as 'victims rather than survivors') was reinforced in studies such as those by Townsend, which depicted retirement as leading to a crisis of identity for older men.[28] The image of retirement in the 1950s was dominated by medical literature linking loss of employment with increased rates of sickness and premature death.[29] In this light, older men were presented as a 'roleless' group, devoid of the moral authority

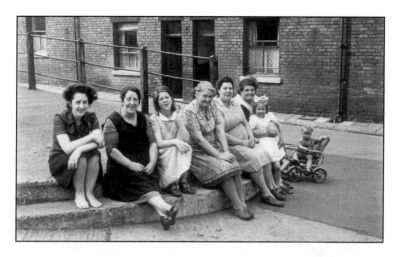

Plate 2: Intergenerational group of women pictured in a Yorkshire mining village in the early 1950s

Source: © Wakefield MDC, Museum and Arts, reproduced in *World Famous Round Here: The Photographs of Jack Hulme.*

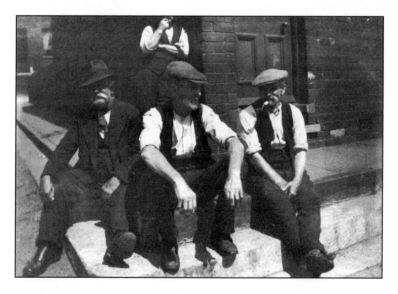

Plate 3: Group of men on a street corner in a Yorkshire mining village, early 1950s

Source: © Wakefield MDC, Museum and Arts, reproduced in *World Famous Round Here: The Photographs of Jack Hulme.*

enjoyed by women. Their social world was to be theorised at the end of the decade as a form of 'disengagement', one which was permitted by society if not by their families.[30]

Yet this observation must itself be placed into a wider context of the hostility of many children towards their fathers, which contrasted sharply with the pre-eminent position of 'Mum' and 'Nan' (a feature most famously illustrated by the Bethnal Green studies). Ross McKibbin summarises different types of evidence from the 1940s and 1950s to suggest that children often described their fathers with a mixture of contempt and bitterness.[31] He suggests that in many cases this was the result of growing up in poverty-stricken households, where the behaviour of apparently neglectful fathers was contrasted with the 'stoicism and self-sacrifice of Mum'. The Second World War introduced a further dimension to the problem of absent fathers. Turner and Rennell are probably correct to argue that official advice to men to avoid talking about wartime experiences – on the grounds that it would serve as a barrier to reintegrating into family life – almost certainly did more harm than good.[32] McKibbin argues from this that:

> The war greatly strengthened female domination of the home while simultaneously strengthening the hold of the wife's mother on her daughter. Wartime marriages were often strangely casual and abrupt affairs – quite unlike the customary peacetime marriage, which usually followed a rather stately courting. With accommodation increasingly difficult to find as both bombing and wartime exigency eliminated much of the available housing stock, newly-wed couples often lived in wretched conditions. As a result, particularly if the husband were in the services, the sensible thing was to return to Mum, where accommodation was provided and rations could be pooled (which meant Mum got control of her daughter's as well as her own ration-book). It followed that boys were raised in households dominated by Mum or Nan in a wartime environment, which normally required from mother and grand-mother as much stoicism and self-sacrifice as the depression.[33]

The dominance of mothers was compounded in many instances by marital conflict. The picture of marriage in the 1950s, as Finch and Summerfield observe, is mixed.[34] Studies by Dennis *et al.* of Yorkshire miners, and by Townsend in Bethnal Green, indicate a significant degree of segregation between men and women.[35] The later research, however, of Willmott and Young in middle-class Woodford, gives a contrasting picture, with a new preoccupation with home, and the emergence of what sociologists were to term 'companionate marriage'.[36] Part of the difference here reflects variations between social classes in marital styles and experiences. The contrast is also with different periods of the 1950s: the Willmott study coming at the end of what was perceived as a period of affluence and social progress.[37]

Youth versus age

If older women seemed at least to maintain some form of control over life, both they and older men were overshadowed by the rise of youth in the 1950s. The distinctive image of this period is less one of contented couples growing old together than of the emergence of youth as a social, cultural and economic force. Young people had emerged as the new social category of 'teenager', with significant spending power. Although some way behind their American counterparts in economic terms, the new British teenagers quickly evolved as 'folk devils', eclipsing from view the changing life styles at the other end of the age range.[38] Inwood notes of this period that:

> Teenage gangs and the publicity they received in the Press and television helped to revive in the 1950s some of the old Victorian fears of London's unsafe areas and dangerous classes. But what was feared in the 1950s was not a class, but an age group.[39]

An exemplar of this was the iconic novel of 1950s youth, *Absolute Beginners* by Colin Macinnes. The frontpiece of the book asserted that: 'A spectre has arisen in our cities – the spectre of lawless, carefree youth. Bemused parents, restless citizens, outraged authority – all show distress at the sight of young people (unnaturally clean and appearance-aware) visibly enjoying their own company.'[40]

In the world of the new teenager, people are 'old ' in their forties and the family is already showing ominous signs of disintegration. The hero of Macinnes's novel describes his own family as follows:

> The family, if you can call it that, consists of three besides myself, plus numerous additions. The three are my poor old Dad, who isn't really that old, only forty-eight, but who was wrecked and ruined by the 1930s, so he never fails to tell me, and then my Mum, who's much older than she lets on or, I will say this for her, looks, certainly three or four years older than my dad and finally my

half-brother Vern, who Mum had by a mystery man seven years before she tied up with my poppa, and who's the number-one wierdie, layabout and monster of the Westminster city area. As for the numerous additions, these are Mum's lodgers, because she keeps a boarding-house, and some of them, as you'd expect if you knew Ma, are lodged in very firmly, though there's nothing my Dad can do about it, apparently, as his spirits are squashed by a combination of my Mum and the 1930s, and that's one of the several reasons for which I left the ancestral home.[41]

Macinnes's description of 'old men with boots and dandruff, and rolled fags with the tobacco dripping out the ends' conveys the sense in which older people were out of step with the consumer-driven fifties.[42] By the end of the 1950s, four out of five families were hire-purchasers of goods, with young housewives a key target for the new consumer market. Robert Opie's *1950s Scrapbook* displays some of the consumer images of the period – Maxwell House, Kit-Kat, Jif Plastic Lemons, Weetabix – some of which have attained classic status.[43] The feel of the times is summarised by Cole Moreton in the following way:

> Ah Bisto! Ah, the 1950s. Those were the days when Mummy stayed at home all day in her nylon 'dress overall', and gathered up dust with a Ewbank carpet sweeper. Taking a bottle of milk from the Coldrator refrigerator – as mentioned in the wireless on the Archers – she made a cup of Lyons tea. There was just time to enjoy a cool Capstan and flick through Housewife magazine before Janet and John returned from school.[44]

By the end of the 1950s, there was some evidence that the 'old men with boots and dandruff' were being replaced by a new type of retiree. The signs for this were clearly posted in Willmott and Young's *Family and Class in a London Suburb*. This study suggested that there was evidence of a more 'companionate conception of marriage', built around the greater attachment of men as well as women to home and household. Certainly, middle- and working-class male Woodfordians were unlikely to be seen loitering on suburban street corners. Instead, they were engaged in developing what Willmott and Young referred to as the 'new cult of the amateur handyman, with the [husband] as busy keeping up with rapidly changing fashions of interior decoration and design as his wife is kept absorbed in conforming to rising and ever-changing standards of child-care, cookery and dress'.[45]

Yet, with the benefit of hindsight, the 1950s must have been a difficult period in which to grow old. The welfare state had established a new set of rights for older people, enshrined in the state retirement pension, and the national health service. But older people were marginalised rather than liberated by greater affluence. The dominant images of the decade were more likely to be drawn from teenage 'folk devils' and suburban housewives. Older people were biding their time before advancing their own case for freedom and affluence.

Urban blues and the rise of the risk society

Moving into the 1990s, we find a different landscape for those who had been the younger generations of the older people interviewed by Sheldon, Townsend, and Willmott and Young. The nuclear family of the 1950s was now assailed by images of division and fragmentation. Ray Pahl observed that, at the end of the 1990s, there is a growing awareness that 'going for growth' with the 'enterprise culture' is not producing a more contented or more happier society. Poverty confronts us in the streets, surveys report people's fear of crime and disorder, and moral entrepreneurs claim to detect a failure in the quality of family life: a 'parenting deficit', in Etzioni's phrase.[46]

The wider themes were dissected in studies such as Elliott and Atkinson's *The Age of Insecurity*, Dunant and Porter's *The Age of Anxiety* and Fukuyama's *The Great Disruption*.[47] Empirical observations were theorised by sociologists such as Ulrich Beck and Anthony Giddens in relation to the rise of the 'risk society', and the 'post-traditional society'.[48] These suggested a new social order of 'high modernity', where identity was subject to major new threats and harmful behaviours on the one side, but offered significant possibilities for growth and development on the other. Growing old was itself undergoing change in the move from a modern to a late-modern world. For older people, this was presented as involving the reconstruction of later life as a period of potential choice, but also of risk and danger.[49] In a post-traditional order, older people had to confront complex moral dilemmas and choices in their relationships with family and friends: a different world from the fixed compass point provided by 'Mum' and 'Nan' in the 1950s.

Underneath the social relationships of late modernity, was the pervasive theme of a more conflictual and divided society, as captured in accounts by Davies in *Dark Heart: The Shocking Truth About Hidden Britain* and Cohn's *Yes We Have No: Adventures in Other England*.[50]

The theme of social exclusion was reflected in numerous urban novels of the 1980s and 1990s, highlighting racism and violence in the post-industrial city.[51] Such experiences – evident in the 1950s and 1960s – had accelerated with the growth of inequalities from the 1970s onwards. By the 1990s, the theme of escaping the city had become commonplace. Walking the streets of London, Ian Sinclair observes that: 'Bethnal Green is a foreign country, it's where they're all escaping from'.[52] The dullness and blight of the city is conveyed by the fictional housing officer in Ben Richards's novel *Throwing the House Out of the Window*:

> Most people who live on the estate are trying to leave it. Twenty-five minutes on the tube from Whitechapel, a fifteen minute walk from the tube station, it is part of a depressing sprawl of estates, hemmed in by canals and gasworks, roads without shops which appear to go nowhere in particular, and isolated pubs which are either called the British Lion or the British Bulldog. It is not a place that is ever likely to be gentrified, since the raw material for such a process – street property – is almost completely absent. There are only a few pockets of small terraced housing, some of which also belong to the council. The most frequent complaint from the tenants is that they cannot move to wherever they want to go because the council has given all the decent housing to Asian families. 'If I was a Paki you'd move me quick enough', they say sullenly when I tell them that they are unlikely to qualify for transfer. 'You've gotta be a Paki to get anything from the council'.[53]

Family life changed with city life. The teenagers of the 1950s have mutated into complex class, gender and ethnic-based forms. Cornell describes girl gangs from Dagenham on a Saturday raid to Oxford Street. The contrast with the ordered world of mums and daughters of the 1950s is instructive:

> They were both born on the same day, a year apart, and met in secondary school where Diz was the oldest and Kiker the youngest in the class. Then Kiker didn't remember seeing her around for a year or so until she bumped into Diz outside the Heathway shops. Diz had grown up from a skinny kid into a tall, well-built young woman, though she didn't smile as much as Kiker remembered. They were best friends from then on but Diz never said what happened during that missing bit of her life. Kiker knew Diz went

to see a counsellor sometimes but thought that was the social services pressing her to deal with her violence, first of all against herself (the scars up her arms) and then against others. She has a violent temper inherited from her father. He's dead now.

Kiker never knew her parents. Her mother threw herself in the Thames near the Docks. Father unknown.[54]

Novels such as Berne's *A Crime in the Neighbourhood* spoke of the sense of moral decay which seemed to run through affluent communities. This was itself linked to the emergence of a more fragmented family life, one full of spaces and separations. The narrator in Berne's novel comments:

> Of course, for many people who grew up in the '70s, childhood was spent between parents, rather than with them. If parents didn't actually divorce, they certainly thought about it, often out loud, and sometimes requested their children's advice. I've heard horror stories about Christmas spent in airports, scenes at high school graduations, photo albums with one parent scissored out. I have heard so many of these stories that they are no longer remarkable – in fact, they have stopped being stories at all and have turned into cliches, and the more predictable the worse they are: the father remarries a witch who dislikes his children and turns him against them; the mother remarries a brute who likes her daughter too much. But any cliche has a fact for a heart, and the fact is that marriages, like political alliances, broke up all over this country in the 1970s.[55]

On a more positive note, the apparent loss of some family relationships was also seen to have allowed other types of relationships to flourish. Pahl, for example, raised the possibility that friends are taking over from given families as new 'families of choice'. Friends, in certain circumstances, may have become more important than relatives or neighbours for providing help with shopping, home maintenance and practical help on a day-to-day basis. Pahl concludes from this that:

> Friendship is a relationship built upon the whole person and aims at a psychological intimacy, which makes it, in practice, a rare phenomenon in its purity, even though it may be more widely desired. It is a relationship based on freedom and is, at the same time, a guarantor of freedom. A society in which this kind of friendship is

growing and flourishing is qualitatively different from a society based on the culturally reinforced norms of kinship and institutional roles and behaviour.[56]

The emergence of a broader range of social relations in the lives of older people (illustrated in novels such as Lurie's *The Last Resort*) indicated a different social world for older people from that of the 1950s.[57] The identities of older people were now being constructed on a broader framework than that associated with kinship and the family. The idea of the 'third age' of activity and leisure had emerged, with a more complex social space opening up after the middle phase of the life course.[58] Older age was, then, being refashioned in the context of a society that was more fractured than before, notably in respect of income, class, gender and ethnic identity. If the fifties had seen a 'youthquake', the nineties were about 'gray panthers' and soon-to-be-graying baby boomers. This observation leads to an important research question for us to consider: does the family matter any less to older people at the end of the twentieth century than it did in the middle? A different family certainly, both more compact *and* more spread out. But is it less involved with the daily lives of older people? Have other relationships stepped in to replace the family? Is it still meaningful to talk about the family life of older people? These are some of the questions which this book sets out to answer.

Structure of the book

The book is divided into three parts: Part 1 explores further the background to the research undertaken for this book, both in respect of methodology and the nature of the localities in which people were interviewed. Part 2 sets out some key empirical findings, in relation to family life, neighbouring and social support. Part 3 explores these findings in more detail using a mixture of quantitative and qualitative data from the research. There is also a concluding chapter which presents an overview and assessment of the nature of social change and its impact on family and community life.

The theme of each chapter is as follows. Chapter 2 examines different ways of looking at social networks and social support. The chapter examines current debates about social relationships in old age, and the impact of population changes since the baseline studies, reviews an approach which looks at relationships in old age as a product of different kinds of 'social networks', and, finally, summarises the main features of the methodology used for the study. Chapter 3 relates our study to wider debates about the changing nature of community and locality, notably those which arise with the transformations effected by globalisation. The first part of the chapter looks at the way in which ideas about 'community' are being reassessed within contemporary sociology. In the second part, we examine some of the ways in which the three localities of Bethnal Green, Wolverhampton, and Woodford have changed over the course of the twentieth century.

The three chapters in Part 2 of the study provide a detailed exploration of the family and community life of older people: Chapter 4 looks at household composition and social networks; Chapter 5 examines relationships within the three localities studied; Chapter 6 assesses the support network and the links between family and friends.

Part 3 takes up some of the findings in these chapters and relates them to particular issues and concerns: Chapter 7 examines the management of support in old age; Chapter 8 reviews support from the perspective of different generations; Chapter 9 views the family life of older people from the experience of minority ethnic groups; Chapter 10 considers broader dimensions to the social world of older people, especially in relation to retirement and leisure. Finally, the main themes of the research are brought together in Chapter 11, where we summarise the main features of change in the family and community life of older people, and the implications for the development of social policy.

In some respects this has been both a difficult and unusual study to write. What we have tried to do is give the reader a picture of life in the 1950s for older people, as contrasted with life at the beginning of a new century. Each chapter switches backwards and forwards from these vantage points, using the perspective of the baseline studies on the one hand, and our own research on the other. We hope that this provides material which allows us (and the reader) to answer questions about how family and community life has changed. The point is not so much whether it is better or worse, but more interestingly (we would argue) in what way is it different? Or still the same? Or just doing a variation of what it has always done through the centuries? We hope our study provides some clues to these important questions.

Chapter 2

Social networks and social support in old age

Introduction

Chapter 1 provided an account of social and cultural change from the 1950s through to the 1990s. As suggested at the end of the chapter, this was a period which saw a transformation of the images associated with old age. But the precise nature of this change is still unclear, and separating the different influences – changing social attitudes, the twists and turns of individual biographies, as well as the process of ageing – raises many complex issues and problems. The purpose of this chapter is to introduce different ways of thinking about the family and community life of older people. The chapter is divided into four main parts: first, an assessment of current debates about social relationships in old age, and the impact of population changes since the baseline studies. Second, a review of an approach which views relationships as a product of different kinds of 'social networks'. Third, this discussion about networks is linked to the objectives of our own study, and the particular methods adopted for the research. Finally, there is a description of the respondents discussed and analysed in this book.

The view explored in this study is of older people with a potentially diverse range of relationships, comprising 'intimate and active ties with friends, neighbours, and [former] workmates as well as with kin'.[1] Traditionally, gerontological research has placed the family as the dominant social group in the lives of older people.[2] This was highlighted by Peter Townsend in his book *The Family Life of Old People*. The conclusion of this research was that:

> if many of the processes and problems of ageing are to be understood, old people must be studied as members of families (which usually means extended families of three generations); and if this is true, those concerned with health and social administration must, at

every stage, treat old people as an inseparable part of a family group, which is more than just a residential unit. They are not simply individuals, let alone 'cases' occupying beds or chairs. They are members of families and whether or not they are treated as such largely determines their security, their health, and their happiness.[3]

More recent research, however, suggests some modification may be necessary to this view. First, as discussed below, changes to the family as a social group indicate the desirability of a broader understanding of social relations in old age. This argument has been conceptualised in a variety of ways in sociological perspectives on family life. One approach has been to acknowledge the growing desire for independence and autonomy on the part of older people. Rosenmayr and Kockeis's description of the family life of older people as one of 'intimacy at a distance' is widely accepted, even if the implications are less clearly acknowledged or understood.[4] In a different way, this position has been reinforced through the work of Finch and Mason, where there is a challenge to the idea of 'fixed obligations' as an integral part of the texture of family life.[5] In contrast, family responsibilities are seen as both variable and personal, reflecting commitments developed through the biography and natural history of a relationship.

At the same time, it is also accepted that researchers should pay greater attention to different types of sociability and support. The work of Dorothy Jerrome, for example, points to the salience of friendship in the lives of older women, and the need to understand the value of forums such as social clubs and religious groups.[6] More generally, Peter Willmott has speculated that community studies may have been wrong to underplay the importance of friends within social networks: 'we as researchers may have shown a cultural bias, laying too much emphasis on sociability inside people's homes and not enough on friendships operating inside pub, club or street'.[7] Beyond these specific factors, however, are more general changes to the households and relationships of older people and their kin. These confirm the desirability of alternative perspectives for understanding the lives of older people as we move into a new century. Before turning to some specific ways of thinking about social relations in old age, the broader historical trends underpinning these will first be assessed.

Population and household change

This study must be placed against the backdrop of major alterations to the general demography of old age, especially as it affects kinship and support within the family.[8] The range of developments are complex but include changes in respect of household structure, social relations within localities, and the demography of marriage. These themes will now be reviewed, with a particular focus on: first, historical trends relating to household size; second, the characteristics of kin networks in urban areas.

From an historical perspective, it is relevant to note the increase in the size of urban households in the nineteenth century, with the augmentation of the nuclear family coming through children remaining at home for longer periods, the taking in of lodgers and an increase in co-residence of different kinds of relatives. In respect of the last of these, older people were especially important, with a tendency (more pronounced in some localities than others) for women to return to live with one of their daughters following the death of their husbands. Seccombe suggests that the return of widows to live with one of their children, appears to have been very common.[9] Anderson's study of mid-nineteenth century Preston shows over 80 per cent of women sixty-five and over living with an adult child.[10] The practice of children living in the homes of older people was to continue well into the twentieth century, reinforced by a combination of housing shortages (especially after the two World Wars), and financial pressures facing working-class families. By the 1960s, however, social trends, coupled with improvements in housing, had promoted the trend towards residential independence in old age. Richard Wall summarises the main developments as follows:

> In the past, elderly women were more likely to live with a child than their spouse. However, with elderly men the situation was reversed. In other words, if we make the assumption that the significant ties are those which involve co-residence, then for women in old age it was ties that crossed generations that were important while for elderly men the ties within generations were the critical ones. Nowadays, for elderly women as well as for elderly men, co-residence with a spouse is more common than co-residence with a child. However, the major break from the family patterns of the past is the much reduced incidence after the 1960s of co-residence between elderly parents and adult children.[11]

Another important change concerns the geographical distribution of family ties. Until the early 1960s, it was the density of kin networks which was highlighted in numerous studies such as those by Sheldon and Townsend. Surveys suggested that this was especially true of working-class areas; one study, using a national sample of households, found 28 per cent of working class families had relatives within five minutes' walk of their home, compared with 18 per cent of middle class families.[12] The geographical density of kinship networks appears as an important feature of the way many communities developed. This is clearly illustrated in the three areas which are the focus for this book. In Wolverhampton in the late 1940s, one-third of older people had relatives within a mile (4 per cent with children living next door). In Bethnal Green in the early 1950s, each older person had an average of thirteen relatives living within a mile; 53 per cent of older people had their nearest married child either in the same dwelling or within five minutes' walk; in Woodford, the figure was 40 per cent; in Wolverhampton, it approached 50 per cent.

By the 1960s, however, there was evidence for a gradual dispersal of kin networks (albeit a stronger trend in some areas than others). Research by Rosser and Harris in Swansea pointed to the effects of this, arguing that although contact between generations was maintained, there was invariably some decline, with increased pressures for those involved in informal care.[13] Their findings pointed to geographical and social mobility influencing the rise of a new type of family:

> The facts seem to point to the emergence of a modified form of extended family, more widely dispersed, more loosely-knit in contact . . . and with much lower levels of kinship solidarity and a greater internal heterogeneity than was formerly the case in the Bethnal Green pattern.[14]

Rosser and Harris saw the implications of this development in terms of a kinship structure less well adapted to provide care for groups such as older people. However, they also expressed concern about a possible loss of reciprocity in the lives of young and old within the family, commenting that: 'It is the inability of the elderly to share their children's lives rather than their households that leads to the sense of neglect and isolation which many of them possess'.[15] And a similar point was made by Willmott and Young in their study of the middle-class suburb of Woodford:

> But help from the older generation is less common in Woodford than help to them. The real contrast with the East End is that there the generations live side by side throughout life, and at every stage kinship provides aid and support. . . . In the suburb, help is much

more one-way, the younger couple . . . receiving much less than . . . they give to parents who are widowed, infirm or ailing.[16]

These developments reflected a number of factors, with demography interacting with changes in social practices and attitudes. Comparing couples in the baseline studies and those in our own, there are significant variations in relation to family size and the average age at which women had their last child. An elderly woman in Sheldon's Wolverhampton study in the mid-1940s, who had married in her early-twenties in 1900, would have been around fifty by the time the last of her average of four children reached fifteen. In contrast, a woman marrying at the same age in 1930 would have been forty-five by the time her 2.4 children reached fifteen. These differences exert a major influence on everyday relationships. As Townsend was to show in his Bethnal Green study, for the earlier cohort, unmarried children might be around for thirty or more years of their parents' married life, often being available to help in the home when illness or disability struck. For the younger cohort (represented in our own study) the decline in the number of children – now compressed into the early years of marriage – combined with improvements in life expectancy, means couples surviving well beyond the period when children would live in the same household or even within the immediate locality.[17]

Social change and the family

As the above summary would indicate, studying older people and their families at the close of the twentieth century raises very different issues compared with the situation fifty years ago. At that time, research focused on people living within what Frankenburg (as noted previously) termed an 'environment of kin'. Moving to studies in the late 1950s and 1960s, however, there is a shift in the sociological debate regarding the networks surrounding older people. Rosser and Harris, for example, in their study of Swansea, highlight a fragmentation in the bonds connecting older people to family members. Or, as Willmott and Young express it, there has been a move from generations 'living together throughout life' to (sometimes) 'joining when parents grow old'. This development has been interpreted in different ways in the research literature. On the one hand, despite recognition of changes to family relations, sociological and policy perspectives still view support for older people within the context of kinship, which is seen as reflecting both the preferences of older people as well as more traditional solidarities. On the other hand, another view suggests a move towards a more individualised family, with relationships based on 'individual commitments' rather than 'fixed obligations'.

Our research provides one way of examining these two approaches. The assumption we make is that the baseline studies made an important statement about a specific form of solidarity or mutual aid, in particular one which was built around kinship and locality. The question we want to pose is: what kinds of solidarities and relationships have been maintained in the same communities fifty years on from the previous studies? To what extent have the social networks of older people changed over this period? Have they become more independent of family ties? Or does kinship still dominate the daily lives of older people in the same way as seems to have been the case in the 1950s? In contemporary terms, are older people supported by extensive 'social capital' in the form of family, friends and voluntary organisations? Or has such capital become more fragmented over the post-war period, as has been argued by David Putnam for example, leaving groups such as the old vulnerable in times of crisis?[18]

To analyse these themes, our research utilises the concept of a social network to explore relationships among older people. This concept will be used to examine questions such as: have social relationships become more varied in old age? What is the balance between different social actors and groups within networks? How do networks vary when different communities are compared? Before identifying some of the advantages of using the network approach, however, some definitions of the concept will be reviewed.

Studying social networks

The idea of the social network has an extensive pedigree within the social sciences, with its development in social anthropology from the early 1950s.[19] Bott's research in the 1950s on the impact of network structure on marital relations was important in spreading the influence of this approach.[20] Examples of the network approach include locality-based studies, research on the personal networks of parents and their children, and studies of old adults.[21] In Britain, the best-known use of the social networks concept in the gerontology field has come from Clare Wenger and her colleagues, who have explored the characteristics of social networks among older people in rural, as well as urban settings.[22] Bowling *et al.* have also used the network methodology in studies of health issues in old age.[23]

A clear distinction is made by researchers between *social networks* and *social support*. Willmott offers the following description of a social network:

> The term social network can be used in two senses. The first simply refers to the people that a particular person (Ego) knows, whether they know each other or not. The second application is more complex . . . the people known are viewed as points surrounding Ego, and the metaphor of a net refers to the links between them. If the links are many the network can be described as close-knit or dense, if few as loose-knit or less dense.[24]

House and Kahn, in a review of different measures of social support, make a distinction between social network as referring to the structures affecting relationships (for example, their density, homogeneity and range), and social support as referring to the different kinds of help received by individuals.[25] Bowling *et al.* clarify this point with the following distinction:

> A social network is defined here as a set of linkages among an identified group of people, the characteristics of which have some explanatory power over the social behaviour of the people involved. It is the set of people with whom one maintains contact and has some form of social bond. Social support is defined as the interactive process in which emotional, instrumental, or financial aid is obtained from one's social network.[26]

Pearlin suggests that the network perspective calls attention to the entire web of relationships, of which individuals are a direct or indirect part. He also sees the network as defining the outer boundaries of support upon which any individual can draw.[27] He concludes that: 'People are not likely to reach out at any one time to all the resources encompassed by their networks; on the other hand, they are certainly not able to call on more resources than are provided by their network'.[28]

The network approach provided a number of advantages for our research. First, it makes no particular assumption about the type of relationships in which people are involved. The extent to which they may be dominated by kin, or by other social ties, becomes instead the focus of investigation. Second, as Crow and Allan have argued, the concept of the social network raises critical issues in terms of our understanding of community and locality:

[We are] forced to recognise the inappropriateness of conceptualising communities in terms of firm boundaries, fixed membership and rigid patterns of inclusion and exclusion. The social reality of community life is simply not like this, even in those communities which seem to match most closely popular images of what 'real' communities comprise. Instead what is needed is a much more fluid [and] dynamic notion of community, one which recognises that some people are more embedded or entrapped in those relationships pertinent to the form of community in question, be this a locality or some non-geographical interest.[29]

This suggests that network perspectives offer a practical and flexible method for studying community life, which considers commitments to localities to be as varied as those encountered within the family and other social institutions. A third advantage of the network approach is that it may be used to explore issues related to personal change. Kahn and Antonucci, for example, borrowed from anthropology the notion of the 'convoy' to explore the effect of transitions through the life course.[30]

Beginning with the initial attachment to primary caregivers, the individual is seen to develop a variety of interpersonal relationships, these forming the basis for what is termed the 'support convoy'. Antonucci summarises this approach as follows:

Many of the members continue to maintain a relationship with the focal person. As the individuals involved grow and mature, the nature of the relationship develops and changes. At different points in the life course, members of the convoy may be lost either though death or through less radical changes. At the same time as the individual matures, experiencing different life events and transitions, new convoy members are added. . . . The term convoy of social support is designed to emphasise this dynamic aspect of social interactions. [In addition] it seems important especially with older people to know the history of a relationship of support exchanges to be able to understand support relationships in the present.[31]

This model of support relations varying across the life course seemed an important issue to consider in terms of our research. Moreover, given our interest in spatial as well as social issues, attention will also be focused on the extent to which convoys vary when viewed in different urban settings, influenced to some degree by variations in social and population change, and different patterns of kinship support.

Finally, networks may also be viewed as providing resources for their members at different points of the life course. Networks may play a crucial role in supporting parents with young children; in securing employment; in assisting or 'accomplishing' migration; and in supporting people in late old age. Viewing networks as resources raises important research questions such as: to what extent do networks vary in terms of being 'resource rich' as opposed to 'resource poor', and is this itself a significant aspect of inequality in a period such as old age? What kind of resources are networks best able to supply? What influences variations in resource provision by social networks?[32]

Researching social networks

So far we have been discussing the value of the social network approach for our research. In this section, we assess the basis for the actual method selected for our own study, relating this to the key objectives of our research. In essence, the main concerns of our research (as noted in Chapter 1) revolve around the following question: How has the nature of family life and support for older people changed in three urban areas over a fifty year period? Presented in this way, our study has three separate elements: first, the nature of kinship and the balance of relationships between kin and non-kin in supporting older people. Second, the specification of a period, namely, post-war British society, and the variety of changes to family and other social ties.[33] Third, the study of older people living in urban settings; in our case people in inner-city, suburban and metropolitan areas.

The research aims to use these environments both to describe possible variations in supportive relationships, and to examine changes in the nature of this support in the post-war period. Our approach will be to focus upon support as a social relationship which is produced in different ways, as well as being subject to various constraints, in the three localities.

An important question concerns the type of network approach to be taken in studying social ties and social support. From the network literature, three main types of approach are apparent: first, the *exchange* question: this exploring people who might have performed a service of some kind for a particular individual; second, the *role relation* question: this focusing on people who are related to the individual in some formalised or prescribed way; third, the *subjective* question, considering those who are nominated as 'close to' or on 'intimate terms' with the person concerned.[34]

In terms of our concerns, all of the above suggest significant issues for our interest in exploring family ties in old age. However, bearing in mind the thrust of the original studies which were the basis for our research, we took the subjective dimension as the key measure for exploring the characteristics of the networks in each of the areas.

Rather than consider a variety of supportive relationships, our study examines those whom the older person defines as having a central place in their life (what may be termed their 'affective' network). The approach taken was to ask older people to make their own assessment about who was most important in their lives, and the role they played in providing support. The method used makes no a priori assumption about the nature of the network in which people are involved. Family ties may be important; equally, other relationships may be significant, serving different or complementary purposes for the individual.

The technique used in the study, originally devised by Kahn and Antonucci, collects information about people who stand in different degrees of closeness to the individual. Data are collected by presenting the respondent with a diagram of three concentric circles, the smaller circle in the centre containing the word 'YOU' (see Appendix). Respondents are asked to place in the inner circle those persons who are 'so close and important' that they 'cannot imagine life without them'. Those considered less close but still important are listed in the middle and outer circles. Respondents are subsequently asked about a variety of support functions that network members provide or receive. Evaluations of the technique suggest that it is especially useful for measuring long as opposed to short-term relationships; and that it max-imises the opportunity for people to participate in the network assessment.

This model will be used to provide a framework for describing the social relationships and support networks of older people in the three areas. The key elements in the model are, first, the personal and situa-tional characteristics of the individual which generate particular support needs; second, the characteristics of the structure and function of the convoy; third, the effects on the individual, for example in terms of well-being and morale.

In terms of personal characteristics, key aspects include age, sex, marital status, income, health issues, and other demographic data. In respect of situational characteristics, the data here include material on the environmental context for each of the three areas, social activities, organisational membership and living arrangements. These elements determine the structure of the convoy and the support exchanged.

The concept of convoy *structure* refers to the network composition of the older person, the key elements here including: first, general aspects such as network size, characteristics of nominated relationships, proportion of kin in the network, intergenerational versus intragenerational ties, and the number of persons of each relationship type in the network; second, specific issues such as capacity and potential to offer support. The analysis will focus on the resources available to the older person to construct or engage in different kinds of supportive relationships.

Convoy *functions* relate to the actual support given, received or exchanged by members of the convoy. The Kahn and Antonucci measure explores different types of social support given or received by the individual, including: confiding about things that are important; being reassured when feeling uncertain; being respected; talking with someone when upset, nervous or depressed; talking with someone about their health; and help if needed with household chores.

Research using this approach has focused mainly on general samples of older people.[35] Our research complements these studies but provides greater scope for exploring the impact of situational characteristics (such as variations in the urban environment) on the structure and function of the support convoy. Existing work, for example, has tended not to discriminate between different types of urban environments, offering instead global assessments of the differences between rural and urban support networks.[36] In contrast, the focus of our work will be on exploring whether the three localities – inner city, metropolitan and suburban – provide evidence for the existence of different types of supportive environments. Again, given the existence of the baseline studies, our research represents a unique opportunity to provide a review of historical as well as more immediate reasons for these differences.

Data collection for the project

To investigate the issues sketched above, data was collected in two main phases. The first comprised a questionnaire survey of 627 older people in the three urban locations. The second phase consisted of qualitative in-depth interviews with sixty-two people over the age of seventy-five who had indicated at the survey phase that they would be willing to participate further in the study; eighteen interviews with a younger generation member identified in their network, and with twenty-three Bangladeshi and Punjabi households in Bethnal Green and Wolverhampton; and two group interviews: one with a Bangladeshi carers' group in Bethnal Green, and one with a group of Asian inter-preters and social workers in Wolverhampton.

The survey phase was based on the selection of a random sample of people of pensionable age, drawn from the age–sex registers of General Practitioners in the three areas following approval of the project by the respective District Research Ethics Committees. The size of the achieved samples in the baseline studies was 203 individuals in Bethnal Green, 210 in Woodford and Wanstead (older people only), and 477 in Wolverhampton. Our survey aimed for around 200 interviews in each area, achieving 195 in Bethnal Green, 228 in Wolverhampton, and 204 in Woodford. The response rate varied from 63 per cent in Bethnal Green and 65 per cent in Woodford, to 78 per cent in Wolverhampton.[37]

Sample characteristics

Respondents in the baseline studies were selected on the basis of the state retirement age (sixty years for women and sixty-five years for men), and the same criteria was used for our own survey. Our research (the Keele survey), which forms the basis of this book, was stratified by age and gender in this way. There were thus more women (62 per cent) than men (38 per cent) in the final sample. These figures are similar to those in Townsend's Bethnal Green study (68 per cent women, 32 per cent men). However, the proportion of men to women in the Keele survey was slightly higher in Bethnal Green than in Wolverhampton or Woodford, because in addition to the survey being stratified by age and gender, it was also stratified by ethnicity. There are only a small number of Bangladeshi women of pensionable age in Bethnal Green and there-fore the Bangladeshi respondents consisted almost exclusively of men, resulting in a higher ratio of men to women in the final Bethnal Green sample than in the other two areas.

The majority (55 per cent) of the Keele respondents were married, followed by widows/widowers (31 per cent), and those who were single (9 per cent); 5 per cent of our respondents were divorced or separated (a small but important change from the baseline studies). These figures compare with national data from the General Household Survey on the marital status of adults aged sixty-five years and above, where 53 per cent were married, 37 per cent widowed, 7 per cent single, and 4 per cent divorced.[38]

One of the greatest changes since the baseline studies has been improvements in the health of older people, a factor which has of course led to overall improvements in life expectation. The majority (81 per cent) of respondents in our study reported their health as fair or better, and this remained the case despite increasing age (the equivalent figure from the 1994 British Household Panel survey was 86 per cent). Even for our respondents aged seventy-five years or more, 80 per cent still reported their health as being fair or better, and this remained at 80 per cent for those aged eighty years and above. However, 20 per cent of respondents aged seventy-five years and above reported their health as poor or very poor, compared with 18 per cent among respondents aged seventy-four years and below. These figures compare with 27 per cent of adults aged over eighty years in a national survey who reported their health as 'not good'.[39] There was some variation between the areas in respect of self-assessed health. For example, nearly one in four older people in Bethnal Green reported their health as being poor or very poor. This compared with 19 per cent in Wolverhampton and 13 per cent in Woodford.

A second indicator of self-assessed health used in the survey was whether respondents considered themselves to have any long-term illness. Using this measure, the majority of respondents reported having a long-standing illness (364 respondents, or 58 per cent) with no differences between the three areas. This figure compares with 59 per cent of adults aged sixty-five years and above who reported having a long-standing illness in the General Household Survey.[40] Moreover, these proportions increased with age (65 per cent among those aged seventy-five years and above, compared with 55 per cent in the group aged from sixty to seventy-four). The most common condition of respondents who reported a long-standing illness was arthritis (23 per cent), followed by high blood pressure (8 per cent), diabetes (7 per cent) and other problems of bones, joints and muscles (6 per cent).

Approximately 3 per cent of the Keele respondents were housebound due to severe illness or disability, with no significant differences between the areas. This figure is much less than in Bethnal Green fifty years ago. Then, Townsend found that 30 per cent of the women and 22 per cent of the men were infirm or bedridden. The Keele survey also found that there were no significant differences between men and women in the incidence of self-assessed illnesses and disabilities. This finding differs from those of the baseline studies, where both Sheldon and Townsend found that women reported higher levels of illnesses than men. The 1994 General Household Survey also found that women were more likely to report ill health than men.

The psychological health of the Keele respondents was also measured using the Life Satisfaction Index scale, an adapted version of an

American morale and well-being scale. This scale is composed of thirteen questions concerning feelings of well being. Respondents were asked whether they agree or disagreed with a combination of positively and negatively phrased questions, such as 'I am just as happy as when I was younger' and 'this is the dreariest time of my life'. The respondent receives a score of 2 when they agree with the positive statements, 1 if they don't know, and 0 if they disagree. Thus a high score indicates positive psychological health and a low score negative psychological health. Results showed that there were significant differences in the well-being of respondents between the areas. The mean score for Woodford respondents was 17.4, compared with 15.6 for Wolverhampton respondents and 13.2 for Bethnal Green respondents (f = 23.6, p =< 0.0001). White respondents had a higher mean score (16.1) compared with minority ethnic respondents (11.6) (f = 35.2; p =< 0.0001). There were no significant differences in the mean score between men and women.

Resources in old age

The relative value of state pensions has significantly improved the standard of living of older people since the baseline studies. Townsend, for example, found that most of his respondents experienced a dramatic fall in their income of up to 68 per cent of previous earnings, and that retired people in Bethnal Green had little more than a subsistence level of income. Our study found marked variation between the areas in respect of financial circumstances. In Woodford, the financial situation of retired older people did not worsen dramatically, because a greater number of respondents had savings or occupational pensions. Just one in ten of Woodford residents reported having a weekly income of less than £77, compared with just over one in five of those in Bethnal Green and Wolverhampton. At the other end of the scale, half of the Woodford respondents reported receiving a weekly income of more than £155 compared with only 17 per cent of Bethnal Green respondents, and 24 per cent of those in Wolverhampton. Women were receiving lower weekly incomes than men. Almost a quarter of women received incomes of less than £77 per week, compared with 9 per cent of men. Asian respondents were more likely to receive an income of less than £77 (24 per cent) than white respondents (17 per cent).

Sixty per cent of respondents had a weekly household income of less than £154. Average household weekly income decreased with age. For example, two-thirds of our respondents aged between sixty-five and seventy-four years had a weekly household income of less than £154, compared with 82 per cent of respondents aged seventy-five years and above. These figures contrast with a national average for the same period (1995) of £196.73 for households with a head aged between sixty-five and seventy-four years, and £153.24 for households where the head was aged seventy-five years or older.

A significant change since the baseline studies has been the increased importance of cars and telephones in the lives of older people. In the early post-war period, access to these would have been restricted to the affluent elderly. In our study, 92 per cent of respondents had a telephone in their home, and its importance in daily life was to be brought out in numerous ways in our interviews. Possession of a car however, was subject to much greater variation: 41 per cent of our respondents owned or had access to a car, but this was substantially less the case for those living alone (just 21 per cent) than for those living with others (53 per cent). There was also considerable contrast between the areas: more than two-thirds of Woodford respondents had access to a car, compared with only 19 per cent of respondents in Bethnal Green (just 14 per cent of elderly women in Bethnal Green had access to a car). The majority of the Bangladeshi and Punjabi respondents did not own or have access to a car: 91 per cent compared with 55 per cent of white respondents.

Conclusion

This chapter has described some of the key demographic changes affecting households and families since the baseline studies. We have also looked at the way in which our elderly respondents were selected, along with their social characteristics. For the rest of this book we explore a number of different issues relating to the lives of older people: what is their experience of family life? How has this changed since the 1950s? Who do older people count as important in their life? Who can they call upon in times of crisis and emotional need? These issues will be explored within the context of different types of families and different types of communities. Having said something about the former in this chapter, we turn now to discuss the three localities in which the older people in our study were living.

Chapter 3

The social context of ageing

Community, locality and urbanisation

Introduction

This book explores the lives of older people residing in different types of urban communities. Three aspects may be highlighted here. The first is the nature of ageing as an urban experience, one constructed around the advantages (and disadvantages) of living in cities. The second is the importance of 'place', especially for groups such as older people who are likely to have spent a considerable period of their life in the same neighbourhood. Finally, the research is concerned with people's experiences and perceptions of change, judged especially from the standpoint of the base line studies in Bethnal Green, Wolverhampton and Woodford.

Urbanisation and community change stand out as important themes in our research. To explore these elements, the first half of this chapter summarises the way in which the idea of 'community' is being re-assessed within contemporary sociology. We then present portraits of the three areas upon which the research is based, highlighting some of the key changes in these localities over the twentieth century.

Re-thinking community

Crow and Allan have suggested that, for a variety of reasons, community research re-emerged as a topic of research interest in the 1990s.[1] First, as these writers suggest, this revival took place against a background of recession and mass unemployment, a situation that made it 'imperative to examine how individuals and communities interpret current economic changes'.[2] Second, locality issues have emerged as important within the context of fears and anxieties about the extent and type of change affecting urban areas. Giddens, for example, has argued that structural features of late-modern urban society make it intrinsically more insecure than for earlier generations.[3] In Beck's terminology, people experience the urban world as part of the 'risk society', an environment where personal security and support can no longer be guaranteed.[4] Harvey expresses this point as follows:

> Space relations have been radically restructured since around 1970 and this has altered the relative locations of places within the global pattern of capital accumulation. Urban places that once had a secure status find themselves vulnerable . . . residents find themselves forced to ask what kind of place can be remade that will survive within the new matrix of space relations and capital accumulation. We worry about the meaning of place in general when the security of actual places becomes generally threatened.[5]

Third, as this quotation suggests, the question of locality has been influenced by a wider debate about the impact of globalisation. The issues here concern the compression of time and space (identified by Giddens for example), and the increased consciousness of the world as a single place.[6] In respect of locality, one of the key effects of globalisation has been defined in terms of the way in which 'people can reside in one place and have their meaningful social relations almost entirely outside it and across the globe'.[7] This may be especially characteristic of some groups of migrants, but is likely to be a more generalised experience among a variety of individuals.

Finally, and somewhat paradoxically, concern with the nature of urban change arose at a time when more was being expected from community settings in terms of their ability to protect and support vulnerable groups. This was an explicit agenda in the development of community care policies from the late 1970s.[8] These were based on an assumption that social networks were sufficiently vigorous to support those such as older people. Regardless of the accuracy of these assumptions, the development of community care as a central plank of social policy inevitably provided a focus for issues relating to neighbourhood and locality support.

In general, though, these points reinforce an earlier argument from Meg Stacey where she argued for concepts and theories that focus the gaze as much outwards from localities as inwards.[9] In terms of globalisation theory, we are dealing here with a sociology of 'space' rather than 'place', albeit one that acknowledges the interaction between the two. Our approach has been to consider the three areas as having histories that help create certain actions and responses to different issues. Equally, though, there are likely to be external influences associated with, for example, globalisation which transform the way in which people conceive of territory and community.

Older people, we would argue, stand at the centre of these developments. On the one hand, memories about place are linked with reflections about the life course; people often order their recollections about their neighbourhoods according to certain personal milestones or rites of passage (for example, houses purchased just before or after a child was born; support from neighbours during a period of crisis). In this context, there is a powerful sense in which people invest personal meanings into a neighbourhood in old age, constructed around what they see as the mixture of successes and disappointments in their life.

On the other hand, ideas about neighbourhood and community also develop around an interaction between histories of place (developed from formal and informal sources), and existing concerns about the nature of economic and social change. The response is invariably fragmented or inchoate, and may develop pathological forms such as racism. But, in the case of elderly people, at least for those who have stayed in certain areas, there is a unique sense in which locality is experienced as a mixture of the personal and the public. The value of taking a locality perspective (as opposed to a national sample), is that we are able to view old age from a special vantage point, exploring the way in which support is produced through interactions in areas with specific histories and identities; hence the importance of place. At the same time, these areas are themselves being transformed by global processes – migrations, new technology, de-industrialisation – which change the way that support is maintained, and underline the importance of space in peoples' lives.

Building on the above points, the areas discussed in our study represent three different pathways in respect of urban change: first, inner-city deprivation and marginalisation (Bethnal Green); second, de-industrialisation (Wolverhampton); third, suburbanisation (Woodford). These may have different or similar influences on patterns of kinship and support for older people, and this is an issue which we explore in various parts of this book. Before doing so, however, we need to give a thumb-nail sketch of the different localities. The three areas have developed in a variety of different ways since the original studies were carried out. In the case of inner-city Bethnal Green, redevelopment in the 1950s and 1960s amounted to a rebuilding of the area, with a scattering of at least some of the population to outlying suburbs and beyond. In the metropolitan borough of Wolverhampton there was also substantial redevelopment and slum clearance, but with the affected population moving relatively small distances to newly-built estates. For the suburbanites of Woodford, the process was one of consolidation rather than change, with a slowing down in the rate of development from the inter-war years. From this brief summary, let us now explore in a little more detail the changes affecting each of our areas.

Bethnal Green: inner city deprivation and marginalisation

Of the three localities, it is Bethnal Green that has been most exhaustively surveyed and commented upon over the years. The range of perspectives is itself vast – from Samuel Pepys in the seventeenth century to David Widgery in the twentieth – all of which contribute to a substantial narrative about the kind of place which Bethnal Green is supposed to be. Pepys, an early visitor to what was then called Bednall Green, is one of the few to have come away with positive memories, recording pleasant meals with friends of 'venison pasties' and tables laden with 'the greatest Quantity of Strawberrys I ever saw'.[10]

The population of Bethnal Green expanded rapidly from the late seventeenth century, with the spread of the silk-weaving industry from neighbouring Spitalfields. The increase in population led to a new parish being formed in 1743. At this point the population was estimated at 15,000 people crowded into just 1,800 houses.[11] Porter summarises the characteristics of the area as follows:

> its western end was packed by poor weavers, the Spitalfields overspill; the east part, still 'green', was settled by market gardeners and a sprinkling of comfortable suburbanites. It leapt from 15,000 inhabitants around 1750 to 85,000 in 1851, turning from attractive semi-rurality into London's poorest parish.[12]

By 1886, when the area was surveyed by Charles Booth, the population had climbed towards the peak of 129,680 recorded in the 1901 Census. Booth found a community in the grip of intense poverty, recording 45 per cent of the population living below subsistence level.[13] The collapse of the silk-industry was the primary cause. It was undermined through cheaper imports from France, and employment was dramatically reduced. In 1831, there had been 17,000 looms in the Bethnal Green-Spitalfields area, employing more than 50,000 people. By 1931, the industry in Bethnal Green was reduced to just eleven elderly people.[14] With the decline of the silk industry, a greater variety of occupations was introduced to the community. At the time of the *New Survey of London Life and Labour*, carried out in the late 1920s, the main occupations for working-class men were in the furniture and woodworking trades, the manufacture of boots and shoes, the clothing trades, and distribution and transport.[15] For women, the main occupations were in the clothing and paper trades, and personal service.

By 1931, the population (now standing at 108,000) was living predominantly in two-storied houses built in the nineteenth century, but with some in the tenement flats built towards the end of the century by private trusts and later by the London County Council (LCC). Poverty was again singled out as a feature of the locality in the *New Survey of London Life and Labour*, as was the problem of overcrowding: in 1931, 6.9 per cent of the population in the borough were found to be living more than three to a room.

The Second World War was to provide the next major challenge, with bombs and missiles falling on virtually every part of Bethnal Green.[16] The area also suffered one of the worst civilian disasters of the war, when 178 people were crushed to death or suffocated as they rushed into the tube station to take cover during a bombing raid.[17] But the biggest impact of the war was on the housing front. Visiting the area in 1946, Ruth Glass and Maureen Frenkel commented on the way in which much of the old housing had been destroyed by bombs: 'Whole streets were knocked out. Everywhere there are derelict sites which already seem to be part of this scene of urban decay'.[18] Conditions inside the houses which were standing were also wretched: 89 per cent of households in 1946 had no bathroom, and 78 per cent no hot water system.[19]

The war proved a crucial turning point in many ways for areas like Bethnal Green. Roy Porter suggests its effect was to make London a less rooted place; communities had to be rebuilt, literally in the case of boroughs such as Bethnal Green. But the process inevitably led to a more scattered population and the eventual break-up of the pre-war social networks. Porter sets the scene as follows:

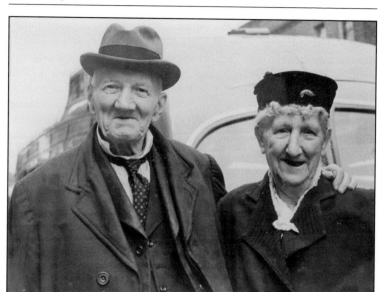

Plate 4 Two friends about to set out to Clacton-on-Sea on an outing
        organised by a club for older people in Bethnal Green, 1950

Source: Picture courtesy of Tower Hamlets Local History Library and
Archives.

Many born and bred in Bermondsey, Bow or Bethnal Green had
gone to the outer suburbs. They often put down roots in the areas
where they now worked. Bombing created mobility. The war
made homeless at least 1.5 million Londoners, mainly from the
inner boroughs. Out of 8 million people, about 40 per cent had
moved from their neighbourhood for some period of the war. In
many cases the move proved permanent. For long, numbers in
London's poorest borough's had been falling, but the impact of
the war years [was to be] vast.[20]

From the late 1940s, Bethnal Green was to be revisited by a new generation of observers, including Glass and Frenkel, Robb and, most
famously, researchers such as Townsend, Willmott and Young from
the Institute of Community Studies (ICS).[21] From the vantage point
of fifty years later, it is clear that most of these studies were carried
out at a crucial point of transition for Bethnal Green. This was certainly the case in respect of population and housing. The shake-out of

people continued fairly relentlessly in the post-war period, driven by the general re-development of London and outlying areas. Indeed, census data confirms that Bethnal Green lost almost half of its total population between 1951 and 1981, dropping from a total of 58,353 down to 29,922 (a loss of 28,431 people or 48.7 per cent).

House-building was of course decisive. Many Bethnal Green residents were re-housed in what Porter rather disparagingly calls the 'dull but decent' blocks of flats constructed from the late 1940s (in reality – as many of the people we interviewed confirmed – they did set new standards regarding space and facilities for their working class tenants).[22] Some people – particularly from the older generations – stayed, but many left. The more economically mobile adult sons and daughters moved out to suburban areas in Essex, or to the redevelopment schemes and new towns in Barking and Dagenham, in search of a better quality of life.

Industry was to change as well. For most of the twentieth century at least, people were as likely to find work outside Bethnal Green as inside it (the 1921 Census recorded 32,000 people leaving the borough daily to work elsewhere). By the 1970s, there was a noticeable drop in the availability of local employment. Holme notes that by 1977 in West Bethnal Green there were between 4,000 and 4,500 people employed in manufacturing in some 380 firms, approximately half the figure for the early 1950s.[23] In East Bethnal Green, 4,000 jobs were lost from the manufacturing sector in the twenty years from 1957 to 1977.

By the 1980s and 1990s, a number of significant changes had occurred in the composition of the population. Tower Hamlets (which contains the bulk of the former borough of Bethnal Green) was the only London Borough to experience an increase in population during the period from 1981 to 1991 (a growth of 7.5 per cent). The increase in the number of very young children was especially important: in 1991 the proportion of under-fives in Tower Hamlets was the highest in London at 9.1 per cent, this being double the national average. The key development for this area is, then, the emergence of a predominantly youthful population (drawn especially from the mainly Bangladeshi ethnic minority population). In line with this, the proportion of older people in Tower Hamlets is below the national average (15.2 per cent against 18.2). Taking the old Bethnal Green boundaries, the proportion is slightly higher (16 per cent) but still below the national average.

Ethnic diversity has been another major social change, with nearly 40 per cent of those living in Bethnal Green now drawn from minority ethnic groups. This has been highly significant for Bethnal Green, where the population has traditionally been more homogeneous than is the case with many other East End Boroughs (see Chapter 5). Finally, an important development has been in the proportion of people aged eighty-five and over, which has increased in Bethnal Green from 2.5 per cent in 1951 to 7.5 per cent in 1991. This clearly demonstrates what has been described as the 'ageing *in situ*' of the older indigenous, predominantly white, population.[24]

As has already been suggested, poverty and deprivation have continued as dominant features of the area. An index of poverty derived from the Breadline Britain survey, shows 39 per cent of the population of the Bethnal Green study area living in poor households.[25] In 1996, a majority (79.7 per cent) of people in Bethnal Green were receiving income support, and 80 per cent were receiving Council Tax Benefits (a majority for more than three years). Overcrowding is still a serious problem in the area (notably among Bangladeshi families). Tower Hamlets has one of the highest levels of overcrowding in London, reflecting the crisis in public sector housing, and the rise in the number of people defined as homeless and in priority need.[26]

In summary, Bethnal Green could be characterised as illustrating the post-war shift from a relatively ordered working-class community (as illustrated in research by the Institute of Community Studies) to one experiencing a considerable degree of fragmentation and social division at the turn of the century. Research in the 1950s provided powerful accounts of a locality poised between two major periods of change. The first had been the Second World War, the reforms which followed bringing, as Butler and Rustin observe, rising living standards and a measure of economic security.[27] Yet to come, however, were the effects of three overlapping developments: the effects of geographical mobility on the family networks of those who stayed in Bethnal Green; the impact of in-migration from new ethnic groups, bringing significant changes to the cultural and social landscape of the locality; and the broader issue of what came to be termed the de-industrialisation of the East End, in particular the closure of the docks and port-related industries. These developments formed the background for our own survey and interviews in the area, and are commented upon in more detail at different points in various chapters of this book.

Wolverhampton: de-industrialisation and social change

In moving to Wolverhampton, the focus shifts from a relatively small inner-city area to a substantial metropolitan borough with a distinctive identity and location within the West Midlands conurbation. The industrial history of the area can be traced back to the seventeenth century when, following the decline of the wool trade, the manufacture of goods such as locks and keys was established. To this was added the making of buckles and other hardware and, by the middle of the eighteenth century, the development of the tin-plate and japanning trades.

Wolverhampton's own development was initially bound-up with that of Birmingham. However, from the nineteenth century onwards it developed as a centre in its own right, with a substantial range of manufacturing industry. Its development was initially founded on the heavy industries associated with coal and iron, and its access to a substantial canal system.[28] By the mid-nineteenth century, the town had achieved a dominant position in relation to the hardware industry and the manufacture of roofing sheets. By the 1880s, a new wave of industries emerged, first associated with the electrical industry, subsequently with cars, and finally aircraft.[29] These were to form the basis for the development of the town at least until the 1960s.[30] At the same time, the older industries were beginning to be eclipsed due, primarily, to the exhaustion of local supplies of tinware, and (in the case of the sheet industry) competition from supplies from South Wales.

Industrial development in the nineteenth century led to a rapid expansion of population. Mason's study of the area records a population of 30,000 in 1832 'packed five to a house and far more in the worse areas'.[31] By the time of the 1901 Census the population had tripled to around 94,000, reaching 144,000 by the outbreak of the Second World War.

Regarding the town's social history, housing – or the lack of it – was to prove a major problem, with conditions especially bad in the period of rapid population growth during the 1880s and 1890s.[32] A start was made with extensive council house building in the 1920s and 1930s, with developments such as the Low Hill Estate, where the local authority was to build over 4,000 houses. But, by the end of the 1930s, the area was still afflicted by a chronic shortage of houses as well as overcrowding. J. B. Priestley, travelling through Wolverhampton during 1933, records seeing 'cottages so small and odd that they must have been built for gnomes'.[33] Brennan's record of the area is more sober and factual, but the photographs in his text confirm the general malaise and poverty that was afflicting the town.[34] The slow pace of slum clearance and re-building was affected first by the economic depression (with one in three male workers in the town unemployed by 1932) and, later, by the outbreak of the Second World War.

Wolverhampton's experience of the war was rather different from that of Bethnal Green, with no equivalent damage or loss of life to that produced by the 'blitz'. Its population had continued to grow during the 1940s, reaching 162,672 by the 1951 Census. Wolverhampton's industries had prospered during the war, with expansion in areas such as aircraft, tyre manufacture and general engineering. At the time of Sheldon's original study, therefore, much of the town's manufacturing base was still intact, while the immediate post-war social change in fact had comparatively little impact on the traditional form of close-knit communities which had been established during the previous century.

However, the major problem for the town remained that of housing. The study by Sheldon provided one indication of this, with about half of the older married couples sharing their house with sons or daughters. Much of this was a consequence of the lack of availability of family homes. According to one report: '20,000 men, women and children are without homes. Hundreds of young couples in the town are living in a single room. Many say they would like to have children.'[35] Older people were also finding it difficult to cope with the overcrowding. Sheldon's survey documented the extent of dissatisfaction expressed about housing. Among the reasons given by those in Wolverhampton for wanting to leave was: 'that the house was in bad repair or that it was overcrowded, with the old people never able to escape from the general turmoil caused by small children'.[36]

For many of the older people in our study, life was certainly difficult in this period, as they attempted to set up home for the first time. On the other hand, jobs were plentiful, with unemployment a scarcely believable (by the standards of the 1990s) 0.5 per cent by August 1950. Half of the workforce were employed in two main groups of trades, mechanical engineering (31 per cent) and general metals (19 per cent). Wartime changes in production also brought increased numbers of women into the factories (notably into general engineering). The influence of women in the workplace was maintained after the war. The Wolverhampton *Express and Star* ran a story in 1951 headlined: 'Dad dons apron to let mother work night shift', going on to report that a 'new family spirit' was in evidence as part of the effort to boost the export drive.[37]

The strength of employment, for much of the 1950s and 1960s, is an important observation for our study. On the one hand, the economy of the area was sufficiently strong to provide jobs not just for the older people in our sample but for many of their sons and daughters, as well as for new migrants from the Indian sub-continent. On the other hand, there was the continuation of slum clearance after the war, and the development of a number of very large estates. Between 1945 and 1965 over 5,000 slum dwellings were demolished, with 10,000 new houses constructed by the local authority.[38]

Migration outwards, therefore, was not such an issue for the family networks in our sample in the way that it was for those in Bethnal Green. The wider West Midlands conurbation, in any event, provided both jobs and housing which would keep people within reasonable distance of their family of origin. On the other hand, by the mid-1960s, Wolverhampton was being affected by industrial changes that would bring longer-term problems to the town. The post-war boom and the accompanying full employment did not last very long into the 1960s. Many of the industries underpinning the prosperity of the area went into decline, faced with competition from manufacturers overseas.

Population change

With regard to the post-war population of Wolverhampton, two trends are particularly noticeable: the first relates to the ageing of the population, and the second to the in-migration of people, from the Punjab in particular. With regard to the former, the 1951 Census records a total of 162,672 people residing in Wolverhampton, of whom 11.7 per cent were of pensionable age. In contrast to Bethnal Green, Wolverhampton underwent a very slow decline in its total population, with the 1981 Census still recording a total of 162,153 residents. By 1991, this had reduced to 153,732 (a 5.5 per cent decrease since 1951). However, these global figures mask the fact that since 1971 Wolverhampton has experienced a significant ageing of its population. This has been not so much a result of out-migration as of a trend explained, at least in part, by the area's post-war industrial expansion which attracted younger adults. The over-representation of young and middle-aged adults in the 1970s is now translating into higher proportions of older people, so that by the time of the 1991 Census close to one-fifth of Wolverhampton's population was over retirement age. Numerically, there are half as many older people again as there were in 1951 (28,516 compared with 19,058). Moreover, it is the 'older' age groups which have increased most dramatically: the number of people aged seventy-five to eighty-four has almost doubled (from 4,290 to 8,122), while those over the age of eighty-five have quadrupled (from 557 to 2,183). Wolverhampton has in fact 'aged' most markedly of all the three areas, with those over eighty-five now accounting for 7.7 per cent of the pensionable population (compared with 2.9 per cent in 1951).

The other significant population change – one for which the area was to gain some political notoriety – concerned the growth of immigration.[39] This had increased during the late 1950s and early 1960s, notably (in the case of the West Midlands) with arrivals from the Indian subcontinent. By 1966, in fact, Wolverhampton had the highest concentration (4.8 per cent) of immigrants in the West Midlands conurbation, many of them living in the central wards and those in adjacent districts to the west which had begun to develop into areas of multi-occupancy. This development, set against a background of relative decline for the town, had already created a somewhat volatile situation, one that was to be ignited and exploited by the MP for Wolverhampton East, Enoch Powell. Powell's 'River of Blood' speech was made (in Birmingham) in April 1968, and was to set the scene for an upsurge of racism in the West Midlands. Peter Clarke suggests that Powell was: 'transformed overnight into an unlikely popular tribune, the hero of London dockers as much as of his Wolverhampton constituents, as the one established politician ready to articulate widespread anxieties (or prejudices) about racial issues'.[40]

These concerns took root in an area which, as we have already seen, was experiencing social as well as industrial difficulties by the late 1960s. In the long term, Powell's racism was irrelevant in terms of preventing a fundamental change to the composition of the population. By the time of the 1991 Census, 24 per cent of the population were from black and minority ethnic groups, of whom those from the Indian subcontinent were the largest group (59 per cent). At the same time, tensions in the relationship between different groups of British citizens have continued in the context of the problems affecting the area.

In general terms, Wolverhampton has maintained its importance as an industrial and manufacturing centre. Only one-third of its residents, for example, travel to work outside the area. But the types of jobs available have clearly changed. Manufacturing industry still employs around one third of the workforce; a drop, however, of around 20 per cent since the early 1950s. Unemployment is now a significant problem in many parts of the town. In April 1996, male unemployment stood at 16 per cent compared with 13.2 per cent for Great Britain as a whole. Out of the twenty wards in the town, seven have a male unemployment rate of 20 per cent or more; the highest in St. Peter's ward where one in three men are unemployed. Inevitably, this has affected some groups more than others. For example, among Black and Asian men the rate of unemployment in 1996 was 25.3 per cent compared with 17 per cent for the overall male population and 15.3 per cent for white men. Middle-aged men (especially the unskilled and semi-skilled) have also been disproportionately affected by the decline in manufacturing jobs.[41] The pressures facing the area have been summarised in a Council report as follows:

> Whilst the number of major factory closures reduced in the second half of the 1980s and early 1990s, there has continued to be a reduction in the number of people employed in local companies as a result of 'downsizing' and the introduction of new technology. . . . New sectors and activities have developed in Wolverhampton over the last fifteen years. . . . However, commuting and working patterns are now much more complex than they were fifteen years ago and this has opened up the prospect of workers from Wolverhampton commuting to . . . other parts of the West Midlands conurbation. Wolverhampton has not seen any major growth in service employment. If anything, rationalisation in the financial sector has reduced the number of offices.[42]

The consequence of the industrial changes has been to increase overall levels of poverty and deprivation in Wolverhampton. Out of 366 English districts, ranked according to the Department of Employment's Index of Local Conditions, Wolverhampton ranks as the 27th most deprived, whilst the weighted Breadline Britain index, indicates that 26 per cent of the population may be found in poor households.

Overall, the post-war development of Wolverhampton falls into two distinct periods. In the immediate post-war years the town continued to have a manufacturing base, with associated high levels of employment, which attracted in-migrants from the Indian sub-continent in particular. In contrast, during the decades since the late 1960s, the area has been subject to pressures associated with a decline in manufacturing industry and a concomitant rise in unemployment, alongside an ageing population. Among the implications of these

changes which impact on the present study are the fact that family
and social networks will, in all likelihood, be experiencing greater
pressures as a result of the reduced availability of work, combined
with the increases in medium- and long-distance commuting to those
jobs which are available. These factors form an important background to some of the issues affecting the families of the older
respondents surveyed and interviewed for this study.

Woodford: the suburbanisation pathway

Bethnal Green and Wolverhampton expanded in part through the
growth of industries within their own boundaries. In the case of
Woodford (and Wanstead), expansion was to come through the spread
of population outward from the centre of London, the middle classes
(in the main) coming out of the city in search of a 'dream or image
of a different style of life'.[43] The early history of the area has been
summarised by Anthea Holme as follows:

> For 200 years until the middle of the nineteenth century, the
> history of Woodford revolved around its private mansions. In
> 1801 dwellings in Wanstead and Woodford totalled only 442,
> mansions far outnumbering cottages. Taking Woodford alone, in
> the same year the population was 1,745. Slowly, however,
> through the first part of the nineteenth century the numbers
> increased until, with the advent of the Eastern Counties Railway
> in 1843 and the opening of a branch line from Stratford in 1856,
> the real expansion began.[44]

The coming of the railway in the mid-nineteenth century started the
process of change from rural to suburban life. By the turn of the
century, the combined population of Woodford and Wanstead was
nearly 23,000. For the first two decades or so, the importance of the
'private mansions' would still have been felt. A local historian who
was interviewed for the research, and who had lived in the area all his
life, commented how as a child it was still 'a place of "big houses"'',
but these were now occupied by city merchants and bankers ('new
money' in contemporary parlance) rather than the old aristocracy.

The inter-war period saw a further spread of suburbanisation.
Road improvements played their part in this, with the building of
Eastern Avenue (Wanstead to Romford and Ilford to Woodford) in the
early 1920s. In Woodford, new house building rose from an average

of 660 per year in the 1920s, to 1,600 per year in the 1930s.[45] The population doubled in the space of thirty years, reaching just over 43,000 in 1931; it expanded by half as much again to 61,623 at the 1951 Census. The new population of suburbanites quickly established themselves in the area. A study of Woodford in the 1930s by the local historical society (itself established in 1932) reported that local societies 'seem to abound', citing as examples: the Women's Institute, Rotarians, the hiking club, the British Women's Total Abstinence Union, South Woodford Literary Society, the Fellowship Players and the Junior Imperial League.[46] This level of organisational activity had taken root by the time Willmott and Young visited the area in the 1950s. They found that while relatives seemed less in evidence in the suburbs, people (the middle classes especially) tended to make up for this through participation in clubs and societies. These, they suggested, helped people to meet others, making up for their newness to the area.

In respect of their origins, migrants to the new estates were drawn overwhelmingly from London. In the general sample of adults in Willmott and Young's study, just under two-thirds had originally come from London, fifteen per cent having been born in the East End.[47] By the 1950s, the area was far from being exclusively middle class, with Willmott and Young finding that of the 921 people in the general sample whose occupational class was known, 38 per cent were manual workers or their wives, and 62 per cent non-manual. The backgrounds of the former were sketched as follows:

> Some of the manual workers are natives of the place, the children of farm workers or brickmakers; others came as children with their parents in an earlier decade; others again have moved to buy their own house in Woodford in the past twenty years. And, though some live in semi-detached villas in predominantly middle-class roads, most do not. There are pockets of working-class housing scattered all the way through the district – the Council flats and houses which manage to look the same in every part of England; the faded yellow-brick houses built for the workers in the brickfields at the end of the last century; the cottages built for servants and gardeners, now occupied by mechanics and lorry-drivers; the bigger old houses now converted into three with a common bathroom on the landing.[48]

Physically, an important change for the area since the 1950s was the building of a spur to the North Circular Road. This served to create an even bigger contrast between the main thoroughfares and motorway approach roads, and the relative silence of many of the side streets with their rows of inter-war semis. As in Willmott and Young's day too, the line of the railway still marks important social and economic divisions, with people living to the east being, in the words of the wife of one of our interviewees, on 'the wrong side of the railway'. She went on to explain that the houses on the western side 'were much bigger and better', while tower blocks and newer smaller developments are now a part of the urban landscape to the east.

Despite this, Woodford suffers considerably less deprivation and poverty than either Bethnal Green or Wolverhampton, with the Breadline Britain index recording only 15 per cent of the population living in poor households. This is further reflected in the unemployment rates, which show that unemployment in Redbridge as a whole was 8.7 per cent in 1995, though this figure was even lower for most of the Woodford and Wanstead wards (the most prosperous ward – Monkhams – recorded a figure of 5.3 per cent). The area is also different in being predominantly a place which people leave during the day to go to work: 64 per cent of employees in Redbridge commute out of the borough, with around a quarter of its residents working in the City and in the East End.

In terms of population, Woodford is also markedly different to Bethnal Green and Wolverhampton. In 1951, it had the 'oldest' population of the three areas, with 15 per cent being of pensionable age. With low rates of out-migration, the area now has an above-average population of older people: 20 per cent in 1991 compared with the national figure of 18.2 per cent. Though still the 'oldest' area, its ageing has in fact taken place at a slower rate than in Wolverhampton. A further point of contrast is that unlike Bethnal Green and Wolverhampton, Woodford has not seen the development of particular concentrations of black or minority ethnic groups. In fact, minority ethnic groups account for just 12 per cent of the total population (with Indians being the majority group). Overall, then, the Woodford and Wanstead of the 1990s, retains much of the 'middle-class stamp' highlighted by Willmott and Young in the 1950s.

In summary, Woodford provides a significant contrast to our other two areas. If the physical boundary surrounding it has been changed somewhat by dual carriageways and motorways, many of its social advantages remain. In the 1950s, it represented the sort of place to which many younger Bethnal Greeners wished to go (the contrast between the two environments being the original reason for the ICS study). Forty years on, the differences between the inner city and the suburb continue to be substantial, with Woodford and Wanstead remaining a relatively prosperous area. In the 1990s, then, Woodford and Wanstead has an ageing population, but one located within a population where unemployment and poverty have exerted less impact than was the case in our other two areas. The significance of this for the social relationships of our respondents will be an issue examined throughout the study.

Conclusion

These were the communities in which we interviewed our sample of elderly people: they clearly vary a great deal as contexts within which to grow old. In Bethnal Green, people's lives continued to be shaped by the pressures and tensions of the inner city, and the struggle against what has been termed 'social exclusion'. Further along London Underground's Central Line, although the distinctions and badges of social class are still on prominent display, there is a more prosperous edge to later life; certainly, a different environment with which to negotiate the transitions associated with retirement and old age. Wolverhampton is in some respects a community in between, offering the range of residential and social contexts characteristic of a metropolitan borough. Taken together, what do they help tell us about the nature of growing old in contemporary Britain? What sort of changes do they demonstrate in the lives of older people over the post-war period?

Part 2

Empirical findings

Household structure and social networks in later life

Introduction

This chapter presents our findings on the household composition and social networks of older people. The baseline studies highlighted the continuing importance of kinship and family life in post-war Britain. In Wolverhampton, Sheldon concluded that older people were an 'essential part of family life'. Townsend reinforced this view in Bethnal Green, confirming the crucial role of the family in the provision of care and support. This finding was also highlighted in the middle-class suburb of Woodford, where despite important differences in the nature of the contact, older people were seen to be as in touch with their children as they were in the East End. The focus of our work concerns the extent of change in the intervening years: what sort of households do older people live in now as opposed to the 1950s? Are networks still dominated by kin, or have other groups stepped in to take their place? Are key network members still living close by to elderly people or is there evidence of the dispersal of children and other close relatives? We now turn to consider these questions, drawing on the survey undertaken for our study.

Changing households

The first issue to consider is the living arrangements of older people in the three localities. Here, the national trends have been, first, a growth in the proportion of older people living alone or just with a spouse/partner and, second, a decline in 'complex' households consisting of more than one generation.[1] Table 4.1 illustrates these trends for our three areas, with comparisons with the baseline studies in the case of Bethnal Green and Wolverhampton. Sheldon's study of Wolverhampton was carried out just after the war and, as his figures suggest, at this point old age was most likely to be spent in the company of another adult. Unmarried

Table 4.1 Household type in three urban areas (women 60+; men 65+)

Percentages

Number of generations	Relatives present	Wolverhampton 1945 %	1995 %	Bethnal Green 1954–5 %	1995 %	Woodford 1995 %
One	Lives alone	10	37	25	34	35
	Spouse/ partner only	16	41	29	38	48
	Other relatives	8	1	4	2	2
	Other non- relatives	15	1	0	1	1
Two	S/W/D/sep/ child(ren)	29	12	24	14	10
	Married child(ren)	9	2	4	2	1
	Other relative(s)	–	0	3	2	0
Three	S/W/D/Sep/ Child(ren) +g'child(ren)	–	1	2	1	0
	Married child +g'child(ren)/ g'child(ren) only	13	5	8	5	1
	Other relatives	–	1	1	1	1
Four	S/W/D/sep/ child(ren) +g'child(ren) +great g'child(ren)	–	0	–	1	0
		100%	100%	100%	100%	100%
n=		477	228	203	195	204

Notes: 0 means <0.5%
– means none
S/W/D/sep means single/widowed/divorced/separated
Earlier figures for Woodford unavailable

children remaining in the household were of particular importance, although non-relatives in the form of friends and lodgers played their part in helping older people to maintain independent households.

Bethnal Green offers a contrast with Wolverhampton. Contrary to a stereotype of the area, it has been fairly common for older people to live alone or with a spouse only for much of this century (Table 4.2). The 1921 Census showed 14 per cent of older men and 16 per cent of older women living alone. The *New London Survey of Life and Labour* in 1929 found 56 per cent of older people living either alone or just with a spouse, a similar figure to that reported by Townsend in the early 1950s.[2] In fact, the major change since 1921 concerns the way in which relatives *other* than children, or non-relatives such as lodgers or friends, are no longer a significant group in the households of older people (in this respect the change in Wolverhampton occurred some twenty years later). This change in living arrangements has, of course, economic as well as social consequences for the nature of the household; indeed, the former may have greater significance given the loss of other income sources such as those derived from employment (see Chapter 10).

The households of older people in the three areas are, then, substantially different from those of the early post-war period. The contrast is between an old age spent with others, and one where it is experienced alone or with one other person (usually a spouse). Middle-class Woodford

Table 4.2 Living arrangements of older people: Bethnal Green (1921–95)

	1921 (1) %	1929 (2) %	1953/4 (3) %	1995 %
Older people living alone or with a spouse	31	56	54	72
Other in households	69	44	46	28
with a child	48	n/a	38	23
in households with a relative or non-relative	21	n/a	8	5

Sources: (1) 1921: Anonymized census data, calculated from Wall (1995) (2) 1929: *New Survey of London Life and Labour* (cited in Gordon, 1988) (3) 1953/4: Townsend (1957)

Note: n/a: figures unavailable

represents what may become the norm in the twenty-first century, with close to 50 per cent of pensioner households comprising spouse and partner only. Bethnal Green, with the influence of minority ethnic groups, still shows the influence of multi-generational households: over a quarter of households (26 per cent) are of two generations or more (drawn predominantly from the Bangladeshi families in our sample). The comparable figure in Townsend's study was 41 per cent, so the change here is considerable but not as great as might be imagined. Suburban Woodford, on the other hand, has just 13 per cent of pensioner households comprising two generations or more.

The major development from the 1950s is the decline in house-holds consisting of more than one generation. Just after the war such households were common among older people, a reflection of the shortage of housing combined with high rates of marriage. Multi-gen-erational households are still, however, encountered as a response to different kinds of social needs, as demonstrated by the following examples:

> Mr Price is aged eighty-seven years and lives in a tower block in Bethnal Green. He has seven children and has been a widower for three years. He lives with a divorced son in his early forties who is currently unemployed. The son came to live with Mr Price soon after his wife died. He now acts as his 'carer' and does most of the shopping. The son has a girlfriend in an adjacent block and sleeps there most nights but sees Mr Price last thing at night and in the morning.

> Mr Park is aged seventy-six and lives in a maisonette in Bethnal Green. He is married with three children. Two of his sons – both of whom have learning disabilities – live at home. One (now aged forty) is very severely handicapped with physical as well as learning disabilities. The other son is partially blind but is employed locally. His wages go towards the mortgage taken out on the house, which was purchased from the local authority. There is one other son living in Bethnal Green with whom there is no regular contact.

> Mr James is aged eighty-five and lives in a semi-detached house in Wolverhampton. He was widowed two years ago and is in very poor physical and mental health. He is living with his only son who never married. The son, now in his late forties, was recently made

redundant. Mr James has a surviving brother and sister, both living some distance from the Midlands.

Mr Pritchett is aged seventy-five and lives with his wife in a semi-detached house in Wolverhampton, purchased soon after they were married. They had two sons, one of whom died nine years ago. The surviving son, who has never married, moved back to live with them four years ago. He had changed jobs and had re-trained to become a long-distance coach driver. He now spends half the year living at home when he is employed by his firm; the other half of the year he spends abroad travelling.

These examples illustrate some of the variations among our pensioner households. Another example can be drawn from the multi-generational households in the two main minority ethnic groups in our samples: Bangladeshis and Punjabis. The Bethnal Green sample included twenty-three respondents originating from Bangladesh, twenty-one of whom had a child or children living at home. Fifteen (65 per cent) of the Bangladeshi households were of five persons or more (a similar figure to that reported for all Bangladeshi households in the 1991 Census). Only two out of the twenty-three households were solo or spouse only, the rest comprising married as well as single children (nine of our respondents were living with married children and grandchildren or some combination of a three-generation household). The combination of generations was also important among some of the Indian households:

Mr Hussein is aged seventy and lives in a four-bedroomed flat on the third floor of a council block in Bethnal Green. He came to Britain from Bangladesh in the late 1950s, living first in Birmingham and moving to London in the mid-1980s. There are ten people in the flat: Mr Hussein (who rents the flat), his wife, his mother-in-law, four sons, two daughters, and a grandchild. Mr Hussein also has a nephew living in the same block. He has three sisters and one brother also living in East London. The grand-daughter living with him was married in Bangladesh twelve months prior to the interview and is waiting for her husband to join her from Bangladesh.

Mrs Khanum is aged seventy-four and lives in a four-bedroomed flat. She is in very poor health with a combination of physical and mental health problems. Mrs Khanum is blind and has only limited hearing. She shares a bedroom with her widowed daughter. Also in the flat are her daughter's two sons, one daughter-in-law, and two great grandchildren. The daughter-in-law is the carer for both Mrs Khanum and her widowed daughter who also has psychiatric problems.

Mr Ali is aged sixty-nine and lives with his wife and seven of his eight children (all still at school). He arrived in London from Bangladesh in 1957 and has been living in various parts of the East End of London since that time. The family lives in a ground floor flat with five bedrooms. Their other child (a daughter) lives in a flat above them with her family. Mr Ali's flat is a converted laundry which was once attached to the housing estate for the use of its residents. He has three brothers living in Leeds, Bradford and Birmingham.

Mrs Kaur is aged seventy-seven and lives in a five-bedroomed house in Wolverhampton owned by one of her sons. The house has an extension in which Mrs Kaur lives with her husband, and a handicapped daughter, aged forty. In the other half of the house live their son, a daughter-in-law and their two children. Mrs Kaur has two other sons and six daughters (one of whom is living in India).

Some of the characteristics of the Bangladeshis reflect findings from the 1991 Census, which showed this group to be in very poor living conditions, with a high degree of over-crowding (see also Chapter 11). Eade *et al.* reported that nearly a fifth (19 per cent) of Bangladeshi households lived at the highest density given by the census, over 1.5 persons per room, compared with less than half of one per cent of the total resident population and 8 per cent of Pakistani households.[3] The situation of the Bangladeshis in fact is reminiscent of the 'family groups' described by Sheldon, and Willmott and Young in the 1940s and 1950s. At the same time, the extent of over-crowding in the home raises the possibility of tensions between generations, an issue further explored in Chapter 10.

Another important question concerns the impact of widowhood on living arrangements. Here there was a marked change from the baseline studies, with the finding that, except among Asian households, fewer respondents were living with adult children; most of those widowed were in fact living alone (an average of 78 per cent across the three areas). However, in Bethnal Green and Wolverhampton, the proportions of households where widows and widowers lived with others was greater than the national average (20 per cent in the 1991 British Household Panel Survey), reflecting the higher proportion of Asian households in the two localities. In almost all cases where older widows and widowers were living with married children, the householder was the adult child and not the older parent (a development foreshadowed in the Woodford study), highlighting the fact that it was the widowed parent who had joined the married child's household.

Changing relationships

Overall, our findings confirm that children (as well as other relatives) tend now to maintain separate households, although this may change with increased age and the influence of factors such as gender and ethnicity. The question next considered concerns the relationship between household members and the social networks of our respondents. Despite the move towards solo living or living in married pairs, to what extent do people remain part of family-based social networks? Is there evidence for isolation among older people from those considered by our respondents as the key people in their lives? In phrasing the questions in this way we were working from what we took to be a central finding from all three of the baseline studies: that the older people in these communities were surrounded by people with whom they had a close and supportive relationship. The question of interest to us was: to what extent had this changed in the intervening period of forty or more years? Some things would have changed: we were dealing with different cohorts of older people with different life and family experiences. But, if we leave aside some of the inevitable differences which arise here, the question we were concerned to explore was: to what extent is it still the case that people are part of a network which is both family-based and geographically close? We have examined this question by asking respondents to make their own assessment about who was important in their lives. In other words, what was the composition of the networks of our older respondents, viewed in relation to ties which they regarded as close and supportive? Had the lives of respondents changed from being dominated by, to repeat an earlier phrase, 'an environment of kin'? If they were less dominated, what sort of relationships (if any) had replaced them? Were there differences between the areas or between age groups in terms of the kind of networks which respondents maintained?

Network size

A key part of the interviews with our older respondents involved them identifying up to twenty people with whom they had important social ties. Taking the 627 people interviewed, a total of 5,737 network members were identified. This gave a mean network size of 9.3 (SD 5.4), with Bethnal Green showing a slightly lower figure (8.3, p <0.001) than Wolverhampton and Woodford. In line with a North American study by Antonucci and Akiyama, network size did not differ between age groups.[4] Although there was a slight decrease in size with increased age, this was not found to be statistically significant. In terms of gender, however, women reported larger networks than men (10.02 among women compared with 8.18 among men, p <0.001), despite the fact that very elderly women in particular are less likely to have a spouse to nominate in their network.

Given the different characteristics of the three urban localities, we wanted to know whether there was any interaction between the effects of locality and age; in other words, was there a significant difference in the network size of the respondents at different ages in, for example, Bethnal Green, which was not apparent in Woodford or Wolverhampton? Analysis of variance showed that there was no inter-action effect, and that the weak decrease in network size was the same in all three areas. Similarly, given that we found that women had larger networks than men, did this finding apply equally to all three areas or were there differences? Again, analysis of variance showed that there was no interaction effect between gender and locality upon the observed larger network size of women respondents in the survey.

Overall, the majority of elderly people could identify a number of people whom they viewed as 'close' and important in their lives: only seven of the 627 people interviewed could not think of anybody they could describe in this way. Few older people (although with important exceptions to be noted in later chapters) appeared, therefore, to be 'isolated' in the sense of lacking close relationships, a finding which held for all three areas, and which may be taken as representing at least some degree of continuity with the previous studies. However, a minority could be said to have only small personal networks. If we define such a network as five people or less, this was characteristic of 30 per cent of those interviewed. Woodford respondents were, however, under-represented in this group, with 24 per cent having small personal networks (the figures for Bethnal Green and Wolverhampton were 39 per cent and 38 per cent respectively). Among respondents with very small networks, men appeared somewhat more frequently than women: for example, 5 per cent of men had networks of just one person or none, compared with 2 per cent of women, and these men were to be found in all three localities.

Children and grandchildren

To illustrate some general features of our respondents' networks, Table 4.3 divides the relationships identified according to four categories: immediate family; other relatives; non-kin; and care-related. The findings confirm that it was still the immediate family which dominated the networks of older people. This was the group of 'intimate kin' described by Townsend in Bethnal Green, and in the classic kinship study of Firth, Hubert and Forge.[5] Our findings suggest that at the beginning of the twenty-first century, this group has retained its significance, still occupying a central place in elderly people's definition of who is important in their lives. Children are obviously crucial within this group, representing one in two of immediate family members. In line with the smaller family size of this cohort, as

Table 4.3 Networks of older people: social and family characteristics

Domain and type	Men n	%	Women n	%
I Immediate family				
partner or spouse	145	(8)	174	(5)
son/daughter/-in-law/ partner	544	(28)	1,012	(27)
Grandson/granddaughter	269	(14)	552	(15)
brother/sister	171	(9)	410	(11)
Total	1,129	59	2,148	58
2 Other relatives	290	15	652	17
3 Non-kin				
friends	450	(23)	881	(23)
neighbours	27	(1)	92	(2)
Total	477	24	973	25
4 Care-related	25	1	41	1
n (named network members)=	1,921	100%	3,814	100%

(n = 5,735; number of networks = 627)

compared with the baseline studies, there was a relatively smaller number of children identified in the networks: the mean number of children cited was 1.9 overall, with 2.1 in the case of Wolverhampton, and 1.8 in Bethnal Green and Woodford. The numerical importance of kin – and children especially – is matched by the way in which they also provided the emotional core within older people's social networks.

Mr Green is aged seventy-five and lives with his wife in Bethnal Green. They have one son who now lives in an adjoining borough. Mr Green expresses as follows the way in which he feels secure in the support provided by his immediate family:

> Oh, I think that family life is 100 per cent important. In every way because I mean for myself now this, I have only got one son right, there is peace of mind, I am under the weather, the wife had a very bad spell and so family life then was, it showed family life you know what I mean, it showed family life, everybody was prepared to, I mean at the drop of a hat they would be there, anything on the phone, I mean my son has got a car . . . and we have got their home phone numbers, posted up down there and that to us is. It doesn't matter what time of the day or night, if there is a problem, pick the phone up. I mean they have got, my son has got us the pre-programmed phone, they programmed them in so that the wife doesn't even have to dial, you know we have got the individual buttons so that all you do is press the button. To that extent they have even put an extension in here for us . . . so you know family life is very, very important.

Mr Barker is seventy-six and also lives with his wife in Bethnal Green. They have five children, and two daughters are still living in the area. Mr Barker suffers from chronic depression and gets support for this mostly from within his family. They live in a large flat (bought for them by one of their sons) where they brought up their family. The lounge is filled with photographs of children and grandchildren as well as various weddings. Although they still have children close by (with whom they are in close contact) both Mr Barker and his wife expressed a sense of 'grief' at the physical separation from their children. As he put it: 'This place was alive [when the children were here]. . . . I mean you go into the bedrooms and they are so empty.' In Mrs Barker's words:

> Oh they are so empty when they go, it is dreadful. After having rooms full of children and their friends, suddenly it all goes and

you think what was it all for, the worrying and the fussing and the cooking and the washing and the cleaning, what was it all for because now they have all gone.

Her husband added:

You don't realise it when you do it. When you leave your parents it doesn't even enter your head, it is only when your children leave you that we think of these things how your Mum and Dad might have felt when you left, you know. . . . And yet they only moved, Anne only moved just down the road and yet the house is empty.

The importance of children was expressed in other types of ways by our respondents, for example among those who had experienced the death of a child, as had Mrs Benn. She is seventy-five and lives with her husband in Wolverhampton. She spoke openly in the interview of the trauma of her son (an only child) being killed in a car accident some ten years previously. Her adjustment had been helped in some way by two of his friends who had remained in touch and who she referred to throughout the interview as her 'adopted' son and daughter:

They live in Finchfield which is about five minutes walk away. It was his birthday yesterday and we went down to see him to take his present. And he phoned up last night to speak to my sister and we all sang happy birthday. So we are really very close in a way which you could say if we needed them they would be here like the drop of a hat. They will come in and make a cup of tea and bring me a cup of you know. [And] he will watch the football with my husband. And they are very [pause] like this is their home as well. So it isn't official but he always says that my husband [pause] this is my adopted son [pause] this is my adopted daughter.

On the other hand, the importance of maintaining a sense of independence from children was also expressed by many of our respondents. This was given particular emphasis among some of the middle-class elderly people in Woodford.

Mrs Lindsall is eighty-one and has lived alone since being widowed in 1983. She has two children who live some distance from her but who are in regular contact on the telephone. Her son has recently moved further away and visits infrequently but she sees her daughter on a regular basis:

I see my daughter once a fortnight, because as she comes home from Stratford where her firm is, she calls and has dinner with me once a fortnight. Or she takes me to a garden centre if I want plants for the front. I don't expect to see them too often, they have got their own lives to lead, haven't they? But I do see her once a fortnight.

Mrs Chater is seventy-eight and lives with her husband. They have two daughters, neither of whom live in the area. The youngest daughter, though, usually comes to visit every Saturday and Mrs Chater describes her relationships with her children as 'very close'. She is clear, however, on the boundaries which surround these relationships:

We don't live in each other's pockets but we are always available if there's something needed, that sort of . . . we're very independent people really . . . I help my younger daughter out with cooking sometimes . . . obviously she's working full-time and she spares time to come here; she's very limited really with her time. My other daughter is also Captain of the Girl's Brigade Company as well, and very interested in the Baptist Church now and so her time is taken up very much.

The overall significance of kin varied, however, according to whether children were cited in the network. Among those respondents reporting at least one child in their personal network, these children formed an important part of it, representing nearly a quarter (24.8 per cent) of the total members. Almost half of the respondents (47 per cent) nominated at least one grandchild as forming part of their social network and it would seem that grandparenthood contributed to more focused concerns around family life. Taking the first five people who make up the core of intimates in the network (and excluding cohabitees), three-quarters of grandparents reported that they had seen at least one of their children within the past week, compared with only 61 per cent of respondents with no grandchildren. Similarly, more than half of grandparents had had regular contact (by phone, face-to-face, or by letter) with their children compared with only 40 per cent of the other respondents. Ties with grandchildren are especially important when they are young: 59 per cent had seen at least one of their grandchildren aged under sixteen years within the past week compared with 43 per cent who had seen an older grandchild during this period. Among more affluent families, financial help in a small number of cases flowed from grandparents to grandchildren, but less affluent grandparents also helped their children or grandchildren by providing child-care for very young children or, in some cases, help with accommodation for young adult grandchildren.[6]

The place of friends

For the 137 respondents who did not place any children in their networks, although siblings, cousins and nephews represented a larger proportion of their network, the largest substitution was in the category of friends: 39 per cent of the networks of respondents with no children compared with 20 per cent of the networks of those with children. These differences were consistent across the areas, although the substitution of friends was most notable in Woodford, where almost half (49 per cent) of the personal networks of such respondents consisted of friends.

Overall, friends appeared as an important group in the social networks of our respondents, second only in size to that of children.[7] Their role may be especially significant in suburban areas such as Woodford where ties with relatives were more geographically dispersed. This was a central finding in the earlier study of Woodford, where local networks of friends (largely organized by women) were viewed as having functions somewhat similar to the extended family of the East End. Our findings suggest that this cohort has maintained active links with friends in the immediate area (see also Chapter 5). These ties are important in sustaining leisure and social activities in retirement, although in many cases (again as the baseline studies suggested), they represent a continuation of a pattern established much earlier in life.

Mrs Hope has lived in Woodford for over forty years and was widowed twelve months prior to the interview. She and her husband had no children but she maintains close links with her sister and with a friend in Woodford:

> Well emotional support I suppose mainly from my sister. People will say 'how are you', and I will say 'oh, I am alright', which of course you have got to say haven't you. I have got a very good friend who lives in Woodford . . . she lost . . . as I say she is one of those that lost her husband last May and although she has got three daughters who live locally, well at least one does, she is one of these people who will do anything for you if you wanted it, if you were to ring up and say 'oh I am in a terrible state', then she would come. She is reliable. I see her every Tuesday because we all go to

the WI handicraft class and we ring one another up. I went one morning last week to have coffee together. It is not a long walk but its just over the railway bridge not far, so I know a lot of people in that respect, but apart from herself she is the only person who I can think of who lives near here. So many of them . . . don't live anywhere near, they live the other side of the [railway] line or somewhere like that. Well one lives, well there is another one who lives near but we mainly communicate by telephone.

Mrs Lindsall has a friend who lives next door to whom she provides support. This relationship goes back to when their children were at the same school together in Woodford and Mrs Lindsall moved to join her friend on the estate where she currently lives:

Well, you see the lady next door, she had a stroke about six months ago and she is very dithery on her feet. She is not allowed to go out on her own or get on a bus. She's been my friend since . . . her son and my son went to [the local] School together. And she was the reason I came up here. She lived in Berkeley Crescent which is on the Langs estate over that way. I was number 1 and she was number 7. Well she came up here because the house and garden was too much for her, and then I said, oh well, I would like to do that, especially as my husband had diabetes and he kept falling down the stairs. I have never regretted moving here because I am in between Snaresbrook and George Lane. I can go on the train that way or this way. I have got a free bus pass. What more could you want?

Mrs Craig is eighty and lives with her husband. She has two children. Friends also feature prominently in her network. She has been a member of the Red Cross for over thirty years, with a lot of her friends coming from this organisation. She describes how she met one of her closest friends as follows:

Well, years ago I knew her daughters, her daughters were my cadets when I was in the Red Cross. That's how I got to know her really and then when her children grew up I met her up at a Flower Display at Korkey Hall and she told me about the flower club and she said 'well come along next month you know and you might like it'. We didn't know each other at all then, and then I used to go to the flower club and then it got to the stage when I used to give her a lift home. She lives in Wanstead, and eventually we got quite close. I mean we very often, I go there every Tuesday I very often get shopping for her on a Tuesday morning, take it in because she's a widow and she doesn't drive or anything so she's glad to have the bulkiest ones taken in sort of thing but er. I mean knowing her has changed my life. Something, we go to the flower club, and through the flower club I made quite a lot of friends you know, sort of casual friends more . . . not close.

Environments of kin?

The above discussion still leaves unresolved whether, as in the 1950s, the lives of older people revolve almost entirely around the family. We can shed some light on this by placing our respondents into different network categories: immediate family (spouse, partner, child, sibling, grandchildren, children-in-law and parent); extended family (all other relatives); friends and neighbours. Taken overall, 61 per cent of respondents could identify a network comprised of all three categories, suggesting an opening out of the social world of our elderly respondents. However, as indicated by Table 4.4, there were important differences between the areas in respect of access to these network categories. The contrast between Bethnal Green and Woodford is especially striking: in the former, nearly one in three relied upon immediate family alone, compared with less than one in five in the case of Woodford. Close to 70 per cent of Woodfordians had a social network embracing all network categories, compared with 62 per cent in Wolverhampton, and just 50 per cent in Bethnal Green.

The findings in Table 4.4 indicate the survival of a more robust social convoy in Woodford, especially when contrasted with the situation in Bethnal Green. Older Woodfordians are clearly not 'family dependent' in respect of the intimate ties which they maintain. This finding may have important implications for variations in the management of support, and the maintenance of reciprocity: does a more diverse social network make a difference in managing the different types of change affecting daily life in old age? This is a question to which we shall return in later chapters.

Network proximity and contact

The next issue to be examined concerns the extent to which those people defined as close or important were also living in the immediate locality of our respondents. The baseline studies had demonstrated that

Table 4.4 Network type and locality

	Wolverhampton		Bethnal Green		Woodford	
	n	%	n	%	n	%
Immediate family	58	26	58	30	38	19
Immediate and extended	19	8	25	13	13	7
Extended/other	9	4	13	7	11	6
Immediate/ extended/other	141	62	97	50	138	69
Total	227	100	193	100	200	100

children and other relations were both supportive and living either in the same locality or close by. To what extent was this still the case with our own sample? Our information comes from data collected about the first five people whom respondents listed in their network. The majority of these are recorded in the inner circle which means that in terms of our model they are the most important support providers and recipients: those people whom respondents identify as 'very close'. Table 4.5 illustrates the proximity of the nearest person in this group (excluding those living in the household). Overall, 72 per cent of respondents had their nearest network member living within four miles. Wolverhampton was slightly different with a figure of 80 per cent. In contrast, nearly a quarter (24 per cent) of Bethnal Green respondents had their nearest network member living at a distance of ten or more miles.

Table 4.6 looks at proximity in a different way, by taking the nearest child in the first five people listed in the network, but including in this case children living within the household. This table also details research findings from the early 1950s onwards where the data is similar to, albeit not strictly comparable with, our own. The Bethnal Green and Swansea studies in the 1950s reported high numbers of older people with their nearest child either in the same household or in the same district (85 per cent for Bethnal Green and 68 per cent for Swansea).[8] The Abrams' study in the mid-1970s confirmed the extent to which children had moved out of the household, but with a substantial number still having close access to their children.[9] Our data confirms that for older people with a child in their network, nearly two-thirds have at least one child living within a four-mile radius.

Mrs Hesketh is eighty-one and following a serious illness the family decided that she should move to the home of one her three children (a daughter also living in Woodford):

> I thought I wasn't quite ready to look for a retirement home, depending on how my cancer was going to progress. So it was decided that I come here to my daughters ... Well my other daughter lives very near as well so I mean she will take me to the shops sometimes, she will take me to the post office to collect my pension and I will go and spend a day with her now and again. My son is a bit further away, he lives at Waltham Cross.

Mr Train is eighty-two and has lived in Woodford since the 1940s. He lives with his wife and has two sons: one living in Norwich and one in the local area:

> [one son] he's a dental surgeon in Norwich. And my other son lives in Snakes Lane just up the road here. We see a terrible lot of them. I mean we don't go a day without one of them, never. And the one in Snakes Lane rings my wife every morning, every morning of the week.

Mr Cole is seventy-seven and was born in Bethnal Green. He lives with his wife and has four of his five children living around the East End:

> One lives . . . locally, that is my daughter. My other daughter lives in Bow. My other son lives in Stratford. And my other son lives at Enfield . . . My youngest daughter works [locally] so consequently we can see her anytime we want to. But normally we go out once or twice a week with her.

Table 4.5 Proximity of nearest network member*

Distance	Wolverhampton		Bethnal Green		Woodford	
	n	%	n	%	n	%
4 miles or less	166	80	105	67	128	67
5–9 miles	21	10	15	9	25	13
10 miles or above	21	10	37	24	38	20
Total	208	100	157	100	191	100

* Excluding those living in the household

Table 4.6 Proximity to elderly parent(s) of nearest child, Britain 1954–95

Percentages

Location	Date	Same household	Same Parish	Elsewhere	Total	Base
Bethnal Green[1]	1954–5	52	33[2]	15	100	167
Swansea[1]	1960	50	18[2]	32	100	327
Britain[1]	1962	42	24	34	100	1,911
Four Towns[1]	1977	14	35[3]	51	100	1,646
Bethnal Green[4]	1995	31	33[2]	36	100	144
Wolverhampton[4]	1995	21	50[2]	29	100	191
Woodford[4]	1995	16	44[2]	40	100	156

Key: 1 Wall, R. (1992)
      2 Under 4 miles
      3 Under 5 miles
      4 Children placed in the network

Mr Martin is ninety-one and lives in Wolverhampton. He was widowed thirty years ago. He has been in his present house (rented) for fifty years. He has two children:

> Ken, the elder one . . . he still lives at Codsall, where he's lived for twenty years. Gill has just recently moved house but it's only about half a mile away from where she was before. She's come a tiny bit nearer to me. Codsall is about seven miles from here, and where Gillian lived before was Fairgate, about five miles from here. And now its about four or something like that. So I, she always comes as she has done for ages to take me up to the Post Office on pension day and do what shopping I need while she is here you see.

Mrs Burton is eighty-nine and lives in Wolverhampton. She is a widow with one surviving child living in an adjacent district:

> If you go through here, through the flats on to Merryhill and then along Bills Lane and then its just over the Bridge. He comes most days. He never comes on a Thursday. He was here yesterday, and my brother and son come every Tuesday, they both come. They put the world to rights while they are here.

Although children were present in the immediate locality, they were certainly more dispersed than in the 1950s, although our three areas varied both in terms of the extent to which networks were geographically 'stretched' and the impact of this on the lives of respondents. We can further illustrate these points by looking at the distribution of the first five network members (Table 4.7) but excluding those sharing a household with our respondents. This demonstrates the concentration of close network members in Wolverhampton. In the case of this type of metropolitan borough, the chance of having at least one child remaining in the locality was relatively high. This was confirmed in our qualitative interviews, where of the seventeen people aged seventy-five and over with children, the majority (thirteen) still had at least one child living within the town. For those in Bethnal Green, however, the dispersal of children was more noticeable. Of the eighteen married respondents with children, only five had at least one child still living in Bethnal Green itself, and many in the group spoke of the difficulties of managing and contacting a more scattered family group.

Mrs Davies is a widow of seventy-nine living in Bethnal Green. She has been living in the area for the past forty years but came originally

Table 4.7 Proximity of network members[1]

Percentages

Area	Inner (n=1819)		Middle (n=390)		Outer (n=65)		Total (n=2274)	
	<10 miles	>10 miles	<10 miles	>10 miles	<10 miles	>10 miles	<10 miles	>10 miles
Wolverhampton	68	32	74	26	80	20	69	31
Bethnal Green	50	50	59	41	55	45	51	49
Woodford	47	53	55	45	65	35	49	51
All regions	55	45	63	37	68	32	57	43

[1]First five in the network (excluding household members)

from Wales where two daughters are living. She is in very poor health and is housebound:

> My second daughter, well she has trouble of her own. She has heart trouble. But she rings up on the phone. But Eileen [the eldest] comes up. But she said she can't be doing it too much. Everytime I phone her up she says 'Mum, what is the trouble again?' So they want me to go back to Wales.

Mrs Hart is seventy-five and lives with her husband (who was born in Bethnal Green) on the ninth floor of a tower block. She first met him when he was stationed in Scotland during the war. They lived with his mother in Bethnal Green for two years before getting their own accommodation. Her husband now has Parkinson's disease and very restricted mobility. They have one son living on the south coast in Frinton:

> He phones me every other day . . . it all depends [when he can get here] . . . he also has problems, its a kind of arthritis but it's in your spine . . . When it comes on he can't drive so he has problems like that . . . and he has also just been made redundant which has put more worry on him. He was at British Telecom, thirty-four years he worked there and when he was fifty they made him redundant.

Mr Pinner is a widower of eighty-one living on the thirteenth floor of a tower block. He has four children who live in Bracknell, Wales, Ireland and Ilford:

> The son in Bracknell rings up every night. Bill in Wales, he rings up once a week, something like that. Jerry, the one over in Ireland, as I say, I can't speak to him until he speaks to me because he is not on the phone. He was on the phone, but his wife kept ringing up home from over there all the time and he run up a bill of over £400. So if he wants to make a call he goes to a call box. Then after a while, I got the number of the call box like, and when the pips go I say 'put the phone down' and then I ring him back.

These examples bring out the way in which social networks vary in their capacity to handle what Fischer refers to as the 'freight of distance'.[10] For a predominantly working-class group, 'managing' the distance between close kin poses greater problems in the context of reliance on public transport (as noted previously only 19 per cent of respondents in

Bethnal Green owned or had use of a car). Even though dispersal of children had also affected those in Woodford, older respondents were themselves more mobile (65 per cent owned or had use of a car), and were generally better placed to cope with changes to their personal networks.

For many in Woodford, geographical mobility was in any event seen as a positive way in which the family developed. Mrs Lewin, for example, had two children: a son living in Colchester, and a daughter in Stanstead, Essex. She also had three grandchildren now living in different parts of the Midlands and Southern England. Asked about their moving away she commented: 'They should branch out on their own. Otherwise you don't get anywhere do you'. Mrs Lewin and her husband had themselves spent a number of years in Australia after bringing up their children. For them, mobility was part of the business and work ethic, one which was contrasted with attachment to particular areas or localities. Mrs Lewin, in fact, illustrates Jerrome's point that in non-manual groups, members of nuclear families within a kinship network tend to maintain greater distance between themselves.[11] She suggests that older parents may be less intensively involved with their children on a day-to-day basis, and that socialization is more likely to occur with peers rather than children.

Frequency of contact

As a general finding, however, our results confirm the existence of a significant network of people still living close to our elderly respondents. Moreover, this also translates into an extensive level of contact with key network members. Seventy per cent of respondents had been in touch (by telephone or face-to-face) with somebody with whom they were 'close' or 'intimate' within the previous twenty-four hours (72 per cent in the case of Wolverhampton, 71 per cent for Woodford, and 65 per cent for Bethnal Green). Again this excludes those living within the household or sharing it with the older person. The extent of contact is also illustrated if we look at contact from all network members with the respondent. Here, around one-third had been in touch within the previous twenty-four hours (the figures for each area were virtually identical). In the case of Wolverhampton, three-quarters (76 per cent) had been in contact in the previous week: the figures were 72 per cent for Woodford and 67 per cent for Bethnal Green. On the other hand, Bethnal Green showed some evidence for the impact of a more dispersed network, with 33 per cent of the network restricting contact to once a week or less often, and 14 per cent to once a month at most.

It is important also to indicate changes in the nature of this contact since the 1950s. Then, older people depended on someone visiting them (or vice versa) to sustain contact; hence Sheldon's definition of a close relative as someone who lived within five minutes walking distance. Forty years on, contact is managed in rather different ways. For example, one in three of our respondents had last been in touch with someone in their network via the telephone. Although, as already noted, telephone ownership varied by area, its crucial role in everyday life for virtually all older people cannot be doubted. Relationships are maintained and nourished over the telephone in ways which would have been unimaginable in Sheldon's or Townsend's time, when the basis of community was seen to reside in face-to-face contact. For older people now, community may be maintained in a variety of forms: traditional face-to-face relationships; intensive communication on the telephone; and, for an increasing number, online communities accessed through computers.

Changes in family and social networks

What does this review of our findings tell us about changes in the family and social networks of older people in the three areas since the 1940s and 1950s? First of all, at a very general level, there are important continuities. Kinship remains, not surprisingly, central in terms of the social ties of our respondents. When asked to name those who are important to them, most people identify kin as being the main group with whom reciprocal relations are maintained. To answer the questions which Townsend posed in the early 1950s, most older people still retain contact with children, and the bonds of kinship remain of major consequence in these three urban areas.

On the other hand, there are differences between the earlier periods and more recent studies. One way of illustrating this is by examining the areas using Peter Willmott's classification of kinship systems into four types: 'the local extended family', 'the dispersed extended family', 'the dispersed kinship network', and 'the residual' kinship network.[12] Of the three areas, it is Wolverhampton which perhaps best exemplifies a form of 'local extended family'. While this may have been characteristic at one time in the East End, the economic and social pressures on this type of locality have worked to fragment locally-based networks (notably for white elderly respondents). Strong local networks are perhaps more characteristic of predominantly working-class towns such as Wolverhampton, which experienced rather less external migration in the post-war period. Bethnal Green and Woodford represent examples of the 'dispersed extended family', where regular contact (weekly or more) is maintained, crucially by car and telephone. The latter, in fact, had caused one of the biggest changes which we might suggest from our study, with use of the telephone reflecting the contact which could still be maintained with children and siblings even at considerable distances.

In the case of Bethnal Green, it is difficult to identify a particular family type which could be said to be dominant within the area. Dense, locally-based networks are still flourishing, at least among the Bangladeshi families we interviewed. Many live in considerable deprivation, and in housing conditions which would have been recognisable to Ruth Glass and Maureen Frenkel in the late 1940s, and the researchers from the Institute of Community Studies in the 1950s.[13] By the 1990s, dispersed extended families were common among white elderly people, typically, perhaps, with at least one child close by (perhaps in an adjoining borough) but with others dispersed around Essex and beyond. On the other hand, there were also examples of the 'dispersed kinship network', with visits from kin often coming from considerable distances. Finally, there were certainly one or two examples of people with a 'residual' or non-existent family network, individuals living in circumstances of immense social isolation.

Regarding social networks, our findings suggest that the persons who are significant to older people are either of their own age (partners, friends and siblings especially) or the next generation down (mainly children). This point is further illustrated in Table 4.8 where we have divided into different generations the maximum of twenty people each individual could list in their network. The table shows that four out of five older people placed themselves within a two-generation network. In the case of Woodford there is a majority (52 per cent) of people with same-generation relationships (again this highlights the significance of friends). Less than one in five of those we interviewed placed themselves within a network which stretched beyond two generations. In this context, relationships in old age are more focused than in the past, with children and friends the centre of attention; the extended family group is rather less significant in terms of its impact on daily life. Of course, relationships extend beyond those with children (some of whom may be elderly themselves); siblings, grandchildren, and great-grandchildren were also present within the family system. This stretching out is more pronounced in late old age (people aged seventy-five and over), where one in five network members are third- or

Table 4.8 Network composition: generational depth

n	Wolverhampton 228	Bethnal Green 195	Woodford 204
Same generation	1,023	726	1,051
	48%	46%	52%
Two generations	738	586	616
	34%	37%	31%
Three generations	325	212	264
	15%	13%	13%
Four generations	35	16	24
	2%	1%	1%
No information/ Unknown generation	33	37	49
	2%	2%	2%
Column total	2,154	1,577	2,004
	38%	28%	35%

Table 4.9 Network composition: generational depth by age group

	60–64 years	65–74 years	75+ years	Row total
Same generation	551	1,378	828	2,757
	53%	50%	44%	49%
Two generations	345	930	644	1,919
	33%	34%	34%	34%
Three generations	100	373	325	798
	10%	14%	17%	14%
Four generations	1	28	46	75
	0%	1%	3%	1%
No information/ Unknown generation	35	55	27	117
	3%	2%	1%	2%
Column total	1,032	2,764	1,870	5,666
	18%	49%	33%	100%

fourth-generation (Table 4.9). But our research brings out the point that in terms of close and supportive relations, most people draw upon a small and rather selective group, with their own generational peers playing a central role in the provision of support.

Conclusion

The findings reported in this chapter raise a number of issues about the nature of older people's social networks. First, our results are consistent with those of Antonucci and Akiyama, in showing that in terms of significant relationships, network size does not appear to decrease with age.[14] This finding suggests that in later life and late old age, emotional ties are maintained and may indeed become increasingly central as other relationships fall away.

Second, as the work of Pearlin suggests, networks may vary in terms of the resources which they provide for their members.[15] An important finding from our work suggests that inequalities within localities interact with personal networks, producing new forms of social stratification in old age. In short, while our results confirm that older people are surrounded by a 'convoy' of intimate relationships, these may vary not just in terms of their number and proximity, but also as regards ease of access for the exchange of support and assistance. This is an issue to which we shall return in greater detail in later chapters.

Third, our findings indicate the important role of friends in the social networks of older people, most notably in the case of Woodford. They appear especially important for older people without children, but they may also play a more general role in substituting for family in situations where other relatives are unavailable. The social world of older people does now stretch beyond the environment provided by kin, although there are still many variations here. The importance of family life still cannot be doubted for most older people. How though does it relate to community life? Does locality matter to older people, in a way which it seemed to in the baseline studies? This is the next issue to be examined in this study.

Chapter 5

Growing old in urban communities

Introduction

This chapter relates the personal networks of our respondents to the three communities of Bethnal Green, Woodford and Wolverhampton. A central concern is to consider people's perception of change: how do older people experience life in the three areas now as opposed to that reported in the 1940s and 1950s? Has contact with neighbours changed or is it roughly the same? What patterns of support are encountered between older people and their neighbours in these communities? As these questions suggest, we have been especially interested in exploring the ties which people have to their immediate locality. The issue of defining 'locality' and 'community' has been open to endless controversy within the field of sociology. However, for a variety of reasons there is considerable value in applying issues which come under the heading of 'community' to the lives of older people. Crow and Allan observe that community figures in many aspects of our daily lives:

> Much of what we do is engaged in through the interlocking social networks of neighbourhood, kinship and friendship, networks which together make up 'community life' as it is conventionally understood. 'Community' stands as a convenient shorthand term for the broad realm of local social arrangements beyond the private sphere of home and family but more familiar . . . than the impersonal institutions of the wider society.[1]

This 'interlocking social network' may be especially important for older people, given their separation from other relationships such as those associated with paid employment. Moreover, given older people's long association with particular areas, they may view and experience social

change rather differently to other age groups. Both these points underline the case for developing a 'community' dimension to the study of
old age.

The focus of this chapter is, therefore, on the ties and networks
which people maintain within the three urban environments. We give
particular attention to our respondents' views about their local areas and
the contact with the people they define as their neighbours. In relation
to these terms, the following definitions developed by Philip Abrams are
useful guides:

> *Neighbours* are simply people who live near one another.
> *Neighbourhood* is an effectively defined terrain or locality inhab-
> ited by neighbours.
> *Neighbouring* is the actual pattern of interaction observed within
> any given neighbourhood . . . Indeed, the term neighbourhood has
> been used to refer to that area 'where neighbours reside and in
> which neighbouring takes place'.[2]

With these definitions in mind, we now explore in more detail issues
arising from other research on neighbouring and, in particular, some of
the findings and conclusions from the original studies.

Neighbourhoods and neighbours

The importance of neighbours has been a consistent theme in literature
on old age. Wenger's research in Wales reported a high degree of friendliness and neighbourliness towards older people in rural areas. She
concluded that: 'Overall, it can confidently be said that the vast majority
feel that they have neighbours around them to whom they could turn in
an emergency and with whom they have friendly contacts'.[3] Equally,
her qualitative data showed that where an immediate response is
critical, neighbours play an essential role, and that crisis help and inter-
ventions are among the expectations of neighbourliness.

Urban environments, on the other hand, may illustrate a different
experience to that described by Wenger. This may be especially the case
in those which have a more diverse population (in contrast with
Wenger's predominantly middle-class rural setting). Here, theorists of
neighbouring (such as Irving Rosow) would point to the problem of
older people being dispersed among younger families, with contacts
being reduced by the movement of population and the death of friends
and neighbours their own age.[4] These developments may be reinforced

by more general changes to local attachments, promoted by the spread of car ownership, longer journeys to work, and different patterns of shopping and recreation. On the other hand, the historical evidence (as well as that provided by the three baseline studies) would caution against over-simplified judgements about good neighbourly relationships. Bourke, for example, writing of the earlier post-war period, notes the widespread assumption that inner city areas were friendlier than estates:

> in the 1950s, residents in an inner-city slum in Oxford who were being re-housed were unhappy about the move because they expected that 'community relations' would be more chummy in their slum than on the housing estate. However, when pressed, few would admit that they were actually friendly with the folks next door. Antagonism between neighbours was common to people both on the new estates and the old communities according to a 1943 Mass Observation report. Comparing Bethnal Green with the Dagenham housing estate, Peter Willmott concluded that most respondents claimed that the estate was just as friendly as Bethnal Green.[5]

Elizabeth Roberts, in her oral history of working-class communities in the period 1940 to 1970, noted a trend towards greater distancing between neighbours.[6] She argues that individuals increasingly saw themselves in the role of neighbours without necessarily feeling part of a neighbourhood. They liked, she suggests, to be considered 'good neighbours', but to opt out of the obligations and sociability of the neighbourhood. Summarising this period, Roberts concludes:

> Local communities lost much of their cohesion, mainly because of changing attitudes towards neighbours. Physical and psychological closeness was replaced by distancing and, in a few cases, outright hostility. Increased levels of home ownership, and the growing importance of the house and its contents, led to an increase in time spent within the house rather than out in the neighbourhood and also to greater social and physical mobility in working-class areas.[7]

Geoffrey Gorer's research, carried out in the early 1950s, would suggest that 'distancing' was in fact well-established by the early 1950s.[8] In his sample, two-thirds knew most of their neighbours well enough to speak to but 'not one in twenty knows them well enough to drop in on without an invitation'.[9] Two-thirds of his respondents paid no formal visits in the form of having a meal or spending an evening together. Interestingly, when asked if they could rely upon their neighbours, 10 per cent said not at all, and 32 per cent to only a small extent; a quarter of the sample were unable to give a clear response.

In respect of our baseline studies, the picture presented of neighbouring is somewhat mixed. Townsend summarised his respondents' views on the characteristics of a good neighbour as follows:

> He, or rather she, was someone who did not expect to spend time in your home or pry into your life, who exchanged a civil word in the street or over the back-yard fence, who did not make a great deal of noise, who could supply a drop of vinegar or a pinch of salt if you ran short and who fetched your relatives or the doctor in emergencies. The good neighbour's role was that of an *intermediary* [our emphasis], in the direct as well as indirect sense . . . She was the go-between, passing news from one family to another, one household to another. Her role was a communicative but not an intimate one.[10]

Nonetheless, Glass and Frenkel in their 1946 essay '*How They Live At Bethnal Green*', stressed the manifest neighbourliness of the area:

> [It] is a place where neighbours can rely upon each other, where there is a special atmosphere of friendliness, of strength and independence. The people do not apologise for their surroundings. They are proud of Bethnal Green and intensely loyal to their community.[11]

And this picture is reinforced in studies by Robb, and Young and Willmott, both of which emphasised the significance of neighbours in the daily lives of their respondents.[12]

In Wolverhampton, Sheldon found neighbours playing an active role in supporting older people, with more than one-third of the help available to old people in illness supplied by a neighbour (although often one who was related in some way to the older person). In Woodford, Willmott and Young found 'plenty of examples of help given to old people by friends and neighbours'. The extent of links with friends and neighbours did however show some variation with age: with 53 per cent of those aged seventy and over reporting a visitor sometime during the previous week, in comparison with 76 per cent of those aged forty to forty-nine. Willmott and Young commented here:

Some of the older residents of Woodford have lost their former friends – they have died, gone to join their own children elsewhere, or retired to Westcliff, Bournemouth or Torquay. 'On the whole we see less of friends now', said Mrs Lambert, 'The only reason is very much because they have moved away'. 'I have only one friend left in Woodford', said Mrs Robertson who is seventy, 'The others have moved all over the place – Pembroke, Cornwall, Norfolk, Amersham and Newmarket'. As they get older other people withdraw from society. Mr Stockman, who is seventy-six, said, 'We stay in most of the time now and just enjoy each other's company. We don't entertain much any more'.[13]

Given such descriptions, how had the areas changed since the 1950s? What was the nature of people's attachments to Bethnal Green, Wolverhampton and Woodford, as expressed in their feelings about and contact with neighbours?

Residential attachment and experiences of the neighbourhood

Length of residence in an area has often been cited as an important element in the development of neighbouring. Young and Willmott, in their Bethnal Green study, noted that: 'Long residence by itself does something to create a sense of community with other people in the district'.[14] And Philip Abrams made the point that not only does 'positive neighbouring' take time to develop, but that the longer established a neighbourhood is the longer it will take for a new 'neighbour' to find a stable place in the network of neighbouring.[15] Our study found that in Bethnal Green nearly one in three white respondents had been born in the borough (the equivalent figure in Townsend's sample was one in two). Many had subsequently moved around the area following marriage or relocation as a result of housing redevelopment in the 1950s and early 1960s. A high proportion of Wolverhampton respondents had also been born in the borough or had moved to the town early in their married life, and 8 per cent had lived in the same district in Wolverhampton all their life (the comparable figure for Woodford was four per cent).

The older people in our study had lived, on average, for nearly twenty-five years at their current address. White respondents had lived significantly longer at their present address than those from minority ethnic groups. In the case of Bethnal Green, for example, white respondents had lived in their house or flat (mainly the latter) for an average of just over twenty-two years. This figure is in fact fairly close to that reported by Townsend in the early 1950s (twenty-four years); by contrast, the figure for the Asian respondents was eight-and-a-half years.

Townsend also found a high proportion (27 per cent) of people who had been living in the same home for forty or more years. In the 1990s, however, there has been a considerable change in this regard: just 6 per cent of our sample in Bethnal Green had lived in the same home for this length of time. In Wolverhampton, however, this experience was more common, with nearly one in four of those interviewed (23 per cent) having been in their home for forty or more years (the figure for Woodford was 18 per cent). Long-term residence at the same address is more common in Wolverhampton now than it was in the 1940s. Then, around 20 per cent of older people were reported to have been at their present address for thirty years or more; and a similar figure for five years or less. In 1995, the comparable figures were 42 per cent and 11 per cent. Eight per cent of older people in Wolverhampton had actually been at the same address for fifty or more years (compared with 6 per cent in Woodford, and less than 1 per cent in Bethnal Green).

Although directly comparable data for Woodford is unavailable, Willmott and Young reported that among couples in their general sample with parents still alive, nearly half had been in Woodford less than ten years, and another quarter between ten and twenty: Willmott and Young observe that 'They had moved *into* Woodford and away from parents'. Among our sample, couples or surviving partners reflect the 'ageing in place' since the time of the earlier study: 42 per cent had been at their current address in Woodford for thirty years or more; 10 per cent five years or less. Despite the evidence for a lengthy period of residence, the age of our respondents means that a significant proportion of those interviewed (28 per cent overall) moved into their respective area in middle age or later (aged fifty-one and above). Taken overall, however, our respondents had clearly had a long period of residence in their respective areas. Given this context, we shall now consider our data on patterns of neighbouring in the three localities.

Neighbouring in the 1990s

In the context of evidence about length of attachment within the neighbourhood, what were some of the characteristics of neighbouring to emerge from our study? The first issue to consider concerns who older people define as their neighbour. Bulmer points out that all studies agree that proximity is an essential and key attribute of a neighbour; neighbours, in fact, are rarely regarded as living further afield than the street, block or apartment building. Willmott reported a MORI survey in the early 1980s, which asked adults of all ages how they defined neighbours in respect of geographical proximity: 36 per cent opted for next door; 36 per cent the same street or block of flats; 22 per cent within a few nearby streets, and the remaining 6 per cent a larger area.[16] Willmott suggests from these findings that the term 'neighbour' probably covers at least three different kinds of meaning: those most immediate; those in a slightly wider circle; and those further away but within adjacent streets.

In the survey phase of our study, we used a similar question to that of MORI to get a sense of how people defined the term 'neighbour', as well as to see whether there were any differences between the areas. Overall, our respondents were evenly spread in identifying three main categories of a neighbour: someone who lived next door; in the nearest five or six houses; or in the same street. Older people in Wolverhampton, however, were more likely to identify with the first of these categories (39 per cent), than was the case in Bethnal Green (25 per cent), and Woodford (18 per cent), a finding which may reflect lower levels of migration and residential moves in the area (Table 5.1).

Despite these differences, the majority of people agreed that neighbours are people who live within a relatively short distance, and certainly within the same street. Given this finding, how many neighbours did our respondents know by name? We asked about those who lived in the same street (block of flats/building) as our respondents

Table 5.1 Definitions of a neighbour

| | Wolverhampton | | Bethnal Green | | Woodford | |
	n	%	n	%	n	%
People who live next door	90	39	48	25	37	18
Nearest 5–6 houses	71	31	54	28	76	37
Same street	47	21	66	34	68	33
Larger area	13	6	18	9	16	8
Other	4	2	4	2	2	1
Non response	3	1	5	3	5	3
Total	228	100	195	100	204	100

$p < 0.01$

Table 5.2 Households in street known by name

	Wolverhampton		Bethnal Green		Woodford	
	n	%	n	%	n	%
None	8	4	19	10	5	3
One or two	39	17	28	14	15	7
Three or four	26	12	25	13	29	14
Five to nine	61	27	54	28	68	33
Ten or more	90	40	63	32	85	42
Refused/can't say	2	0.9	6	4	2	1
Totals	228	100	195	100	204	100

$p < 0.01$

(Table 5.2). There were in fact relatively few differences between the areas, with two-thirds saying that they knew five or more households in their street; 38 per cent knew ten or more neighbours. A minority of respondents claimed not to know anyone by name. This was slightly more the case in Bethnal Green, where one in ten of those interviewed knew *nobody* by name, and a further 14 per cent just one or two people. Overall, white respondents knew substantially more neighbours than those from minority ethnic groups, which almost certainly reflects differences in factors such as length of residence and general experiences of the area (discussed in this chapter).

Contact with neighbours

National surveys such as the *General Household Survey* show high levels of contact between older people and their neighbours. The 1995 survey reported that 79 per cent of people aged sixty-five and over talked at least once a week to neighbours, with similar proportions recorded for men and women.[17] Findings from our survey are similar to these (Table 5.3). Our question asked whether respondents had talked to anyone in their street in the past month rather than week. There was a clear contrast here between inner-city Bethnal Green, where one in three respondents had talked with no neighbours at all or just one or two, compared with around one in ten in Woodford (the figure for Wolverhampton was 29 per cent). Bethnal Green, in fact, had responses at both extremes, with a higher proportion than in the other two areas (13 per cent) reporting contact with twenty or more people.

A rather more revealing question in terms of contacts with neighbours concerns whether they actually came into the respondent's home.

Table 5.3 Neighbours talked to in the past month

| | Wolverhampton | | Bethnal Green | | Woodford | |
	n	%	n	%	n	%
None	26	11	31	16	9	4
One or two	41	18	35	18	16	8
Three or four	37	16	26	13	41	20
Five to nine	54	24	46	24	73	36
Ten to fourteen	35	15	23	12	40	20
Fifteen to nineteen	15	7	7	4	10	5
Twenty+	19	8	25	13	14	7
Can't say	1	0.4	2	1	1	1
Totals	228	100	195	100	204	100

$p < 0.01$

Regular contact with people on the street is one thing; inviting people into your home indicates a closer relationship, one which may involve reciprocal ties in some form or another. In fact, contact between neighbours may always have been subject to fairly strict limitations. In Bethnal Green, in the early 1950s, Townsend found nearly two-thirds of his respondents saying that they did not go regularly into the home of a neighbour, and nor did a neighbour visit them. And some of Willmott and Young's working-class respondents in Woodford expressed fairly strong views against allowing non-relatives into their home.

Our study asked whether anybody in the street had come into the respondent's home in the past six months. Overall, nearly 70 per cent of those interviewed had invited a neighbour into their home, with the Woodford sample having the highest rates (75 per cent), followed by Wolverhampton (72 per cent), and Bethnal Green (61 per cent). There were some social class differences on this issue. Overall, middle-class respondents were more likely to have had neighbours in their home in Woodford and Wolverhampton (but not in Bethnal Green) where there were no social class differences. There were no significant gender, age or ethnic differences on this issue.

We also asked respondents whether they thought of anyone living in their street as a 'friend'. This was important in the light of evidence about neighbours offering short-term or emergency help to older people, assistance which may be more likely where people are friends. In fact, over one-third (38 per cent) of those interviewed in Bethnal Green were unable to identify anyone in their street as a friend (the equivalent figures for Wolverhampton and Woodford were 26 per cent and 32 per cent respectively). There were no significant differences on this question when controlling for age, gender, social class and ethnicity.

Experiences of the neighbourhood

So far this chapter has focused on questions about the extent of contacts with neighbours. However, we also asked respondents how they felt about their environment: what did they like or dislike about living in the area? How would people feel if they had to move from the area? These questions were asked partly to provide a contrast with the earlier studies; partly, also, to provide a context for the information about the social networks gleaned from the survey.

The first question we asked was whether there was anything people particularly liked about living in their area. Overall, 79 per cent could find something to like, with the highest proportions in Woodford (87 per cent) and Wolverhampton (86 per cent); the figure for Bethnal Green was 65 per cent. Many respondents felt they lived in a friendly area and that there was a 'community feeling' to where they lived:

> Everybody is fairly friendly, look after each other's interests. We have a neighbourhood watch going (Wolverhampton, seventy year old man, married).

> I feel that it is a community. I feel at ease walking around (Wolverhampton, sixty-four year old woman, married).

> It's the East End and I like the East End. I've loved Bethnal Green ever since I've lived here. I've got so many friends here. It's a real community (Bethnal Green, seventy year old man, widowed).

> I think it's . . . I feel happy . . . the surroundings . . . everyone seems friendly here (Bethnal Green, sixty-four year old woman, divorced).

> More like a village. Everybody knows everyone else. It is very friendly (Woodford, sixty year old woman, married).

> I like the position of it. It is a very friendly, helpful neighbourhood (Woodford, eighty-one year old woman, widowed).

Neighbours were also valued, though in some instances for respecting distance and not causing trouble:

I keep myself to myself. People leave me alone and that suits me (Bethnal Green, eighty-three year old man, married).

I like my home. I'm a person who likes to keep to myself. I've got neighbours I speak to but that's all (Bethnal Green, sixty-one year old woman, widowed).

Neighbours are quiet and I don't like any trouble (Bethnal Green, sixty-three year old man, married).

Everyone minds their own business – can live in peace (Woodford, ninety-three year old woman, widowed).

I've get friendly neighbours . . . but I don't know their names. I think I've seen them once or twice but they're all very nice (Woodford, sixty-five year old woman, married).

It's nice and quite and no aggro. We've got good neighbours, and

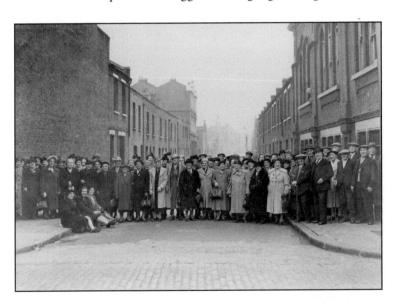

Plate 5: Group photograph of members of Friends Hall Older People's Club (Bethnal Green), taken just before an outing to Southend, 1952

Source: Picture courtesy of Tower Hamlets Local History Library and Archives.

they mind their own business (Wolverhampton, sixty-five year old woman, married).

In the 1950s, Townsend, and Young and Willmott, emphasised the sense of identification which many people had with Bethnal Green. Two of Young and Willmott's respondents expressed it thus:

Well, you're born into it, aren't you? You grow up here. I don't think I'd like to live anywhere else. Both my husband and I were born here and have lived here all our lives.

Your asking me what I think of Bethnal Green is like asking a countryman what he thinks of the country. You understand what I mean? Well, I've always lived here, I'm contented. I suppose when you've always lived here you like it.

In line with these comments, Bethnal Green respondents were rather more likely than those in the other localities to stress their sense of having 'roots' in the area. The following comments are typical of this feeling:

It's my home, my roots are here now. It's what I'm used to living here and working here for so many years (seventy-six year old woman, widowed).

Having lived here all my life I don't know any different. My roots are here (seventy-six year old woman, single).

It's where I was brought up. I wouldn't want to live anywhere else. All my friends are here and I wouldn't know anyone anywhere else (sixty-seven year old man widowed).

If a sense of identity with the East End was important for many of those in Bethnal Green, in Woodford advantages were often put in terms of the 'selectivity' of the area. The earlier Woodford study was carried out in the late 1950s, and issues relating to social class were a prominent feature of the research. In particular, it highlighted the importance which the middle-class in Woodford attached to differentiating themselves from those in the East End. As Willmott and Young put it:

If social class has an edge in Woodford, it is partly because so many people come from the East End. 'We don't tell people we come from Bethnal Green', said one woman, 'you get the scum of the earth there'. Mr Barber said, 'The East End is a different class altogether – people there call you Dad or Uncle or Auntie. We don't get any of that here.[18]

These attitudes were certainly replayed by some of our respondents, albeit with a contemporary gloss:

It's always been considered a 'number one' spot. It's full of people who are quite well off. We don't have many one-parent families here (seventy-four year old man, married).

I've always liked it but I'm a private person and I think this area has a bit of class (seventy-eight year old woman, married).

I like living in Woodford Green as I came from East London and this is a very quiet area as opposed to the noise of London.

Nice green area. People are friendly. Mostly house owners (sixty-six year old woman, widowed).

It's rather select. Plenty of greenery. Local to everything (seventy-eight year old man, single).

Perceptions of the environment

If most people could find something to like about their area, our respondents were rather more divided about whether there was anything to dislike. Overall, 52 per cent highlighted some aspect which concerned them, although this was much more the case in Bethnal Green (64 per cent) than in Woodford (46 per cent) or Wolverhampton (48 per cent). The issues that people raised about their local area showed some variation, although there were overlapping concerns. Some of the responses reflected developments which Roberts identified in her study of three Lancashire communities. She found 'a new development, still only observable in a small minority of areas: neighbours' property was abused and rights ignored. Neighbours were regarded with neither "distant cordiality" nor effortless "sociability" but with outright hostility. The neighbour was now the enemy.'[19] This observation is important given the traditional role allocated to neighbours of older people: neighbours are (or should be) friendly (indeed the terms 'friend' and 'neighbour' are treated as synonymous in many studies). Neighbours help in 'emergencies'; are those to whom older people turn when relatives are unavailable. In reality, however, for a number of people in our survey, the experience of the neighbourhood was rather different. They did not seem to be surrounded by people with whom 'they had friendly contacts'. Neighbours now seemed potentially hostile: a view expressed with particular vigour by some of the older women in our study:

> Neighbours . . . noisy, language terrible, possibly vermin from next door because of the rubbish (Wolverhampton, sixty year old woman, married).

> People don't like doing for you . . . people don't bother they don't. Now everybody's got cars and you don't see people to talk to. I'm eighty-one now. I've just booked into a [residential] home but I don't want to go yet (Wolverhampton, eighty-one year old woman, widowed).

> The neighbour used my washing lines. I told her not to. She ignored. Got my home help to cut my lines down. If I can't use them she is not going to use them. Kids come into my garden – one said 'I'll play wherever I want to'. It was a lot quieter where I was before (Wolverhampton, sixty year old woman, married).

> Terrible with the neighbours . . . they've broke my windows. They are on the rough side (Bethnal Green, seventy-two year old woman, single).

> Well . . . there is a house opposite that has a lot of those one-parent families and the children come into our gardens here. That's why I'm glad we're on the first floor, because nobody can look in! (Woodford, seventy-four year old woman, married).

For a number of respondents, the problems they faced reflected the death or moving away of old neighbours; perhaps inevitably those replacing them – especially if young – were seen as bringing different values and attitudes:

> It has 'gone down'. There were elderly people about our age but

they are all young now (Wolverhampton, eighty-three year old man, married).

Got no friends here now . . . most of them have died. It's not very friendly here (Wolverhampton, seventy year old woman, widowed).

Not a friendly atmosphere . . . nobody wants to know you (Wolverhampton, sixty-six year old man, married).

Some of the new tenants I am not keen on . . . the younger ones (Wolverhampton, eighty year old woman, widowed).

Miss the neighbours – some have moved away or died, otherwise nothing against it (Bethnal Green, seventy-six year old woman, widowed).

The neighbours – they let their children run riot. They kick balls around and slam doors (Bethnal Green, seventy year old man, married).

For elderly people, problems with neighbours merged with more general dislikes about the environment in which they lived. People had a sense of being 'shut in', or that the area had 'gone down', or that they felt 'threatened' on the streets, or that the place was just 'filthy':

One thing is the kids make the lifts dirty. The water doesn't run away in the balcony. There are a lot of pigeons and muck from them. We have cockroaches and rats and mice. I had a nervous breakdown because of it. And broken pavements . . . I have fallen down six or seven times. It's disgusting (Bethnal Green, seventy-four year old woman, divorced).

It's gradually gone down. When we first came it was nice but not now. You can't seem to get anything done. My windows are falling apart and my roof leaks. It seems to be just pieces of paper flying around (Bethnal Green, sixty-four year old woman, married).

The locality has gone down. You're in the heart of the slums . . . You can't do the shopping you used to locally. When we walk through the gate at the end we are faced with lots of rubbish put outside. My grandchildren don't even like coming to visit us (Bethnal Green, sixty-five year old married woman).

Everything seems on top of you . . . you are too compact. Everybody seems on top of one another. Too many people live in a space all on top of you (Bethnal Green, seventy-four year old woman, married).

This flat. I've got no outlet. I've no balcony where I can put a chair out, I can't move out of the flat, I feel closed in (Bethnal Green, eighty-eight year old woman, married).

The vandalism . . . I've got graffiti up the stairs and the lift door, the people aren't as nice and clean . . . there's lots of children and it's not as quiet as it used to be (Wolverhampton, sixty-eight year old woman, single).

One way of looking at people's concern about their neighbourhood is to ask them how they feel about going out alone during the day or at night. This type of question is asked in the British Crime Survey in the form: 'How safe do you feel walking alone in this area after dark?' Respondents are also asked how frequently they went out after dark.

In our survey, respondents were asked: 'Do you ever go out alone during the day/alone at night?' If the answer was 'no', people were asked to state the reasons why. In our study, a majority of those interviewed claimed not to go out alone at night: 70 per cent overall (72 per cent in Bethnal Green; 72 per cent in Wolverhampton; and 66 per cent in Woodford). One in three respondents gave the reasons for this in terms of not 'feeling safe', 'being scared', or 'fearing crime'. In addition, sixteen respondents cited personal experiences of being the victim of crimes such as mugging; ninety-four people said there was no need for them to go out at night; and fifty-seven that they had an illness or disability which prevented them; five cited a fear of racial harassment.

Some of the fears behind these figures were expressed particularly acutely by some of the Bethnal Green respondents, when commenting on aspects of the area which they disliked:

All this disruption . . . crime. Little while ago had a shooting [which] upset us. The area . . . not very nice – can't put my finger on it just don't like it (eighty-two year old woman, married).

The dirt and filth in the streets and I am worried about the crime in the area . . . I've only just been burgled (seventy-nine year old woman, widowed).

I have got the fear of being victimised for many reasons.. I think.. there are violent incidents in the area (seventy-one year old man, married).

We consistently get harassed by white as well as black people . . . Our shopping gets taken away . . . we get verbal abuse and threats. We don't feel safe at all when we go out (sixty-nine year old man, married).

It's not a safe area anymore . . . not safe to walk around . . . and immigrants changed for worse in last ten years . . . [you] do not feel at ease anymore (sixty-eight year old woman, single).

Racism in the three areas

The last comment reflects the way in which a number of the white respondents linked changes to their area with issues connected with race and ethnicity. The extent of racism in Bethnal Green has been observed in a number of studies. Drawing on Cohen's work in social anthropology, Cornwell argued that communities were constructed through the drawing of boundaries between 'insiders' and 'outsiders', with ethnic origin central to the development of processes of 'in-clusion and ex-clusion'.[20] In our study, it is clear that such distinctions are still important, but have undoubtedly been sharpened by the growth of inequalities since the early 1980s. Overall, when asked what they disliked about the area, around one in three white older people respondents in the Bethnal Green sample made explicit reference to minority ethnic groups:

Since the war it's all changed . . . we're getting too many coloured people, blacks, Asians, Turks, Cypriots. It's getting out of hand. They want the law to suit themselves – there aren't any in Ireland where my son lives. In the old days no one feared being mugged or broken into (eighty-one year old man, widowed).

I don't like the way it's changed . . . it used to be typically Jewish when I moved here. Now there is Bangladeshis I think they are . . . they spit on the stairs and don't teach their children properly (seventy-two year old woman, married).

The only thing now about Bethnal Green is that the ethnics are taking over . . . this bit of Bethnal Green is losing its identity (seventy-seven year old man, married).

I got mugged on the stairs. I used to like Bethnal Green but when I got mugged it turned me against it. There are too many Pakistanis around (seventy-one year old woman, widowed).

All the Asians – it's like Bangladesh. We all lived in one street and all the Asians came here and got preference for everything. Now they have all the best houses and gardens which we never had. We were born here (sixty-seven year old man, married).

Such feelings were also articulated in the other localities, albeit by smaller numbers of respondents:

Overrun with Asians . . . they don't bother us but they do what they want and never mind anyone else . . . it's not like it used to be (Wolverhampton, seventy year old woman, married).

I would rather live among white people . . . there are very few here (Wolverhampton, eighty-three year old woman, married).

Too many blacks living in the district now . . . I'm not a racist but it's always been a white area (Woodford, seventy-four year old man, married).

Of course, the sense of threat and insecurity affects a range of groups in the area, and Black and Asian older people will themselves absorb the hostility and incomprehension of those around them. The following comments from the survey are suggestive:

It's a lonely right wing Tory area, politically right wing area, as a black woman it is difficult to make friends (Wolverhampton, sixty-three year old woman, married).

Discrimination. I'm always a bloody Pole, even though I've lived here so long. They always call me a bloody Pole when I talk to anyone here (Bethnal Green, seventy-one year old man, single).

I am living surrounded by racist people, can't go out because of them. I don't feel safe. They don't like me to live here (Bethnal Green, sixty-nine year old man, married).

Many of these comments need to be related to more general problems older people faced within these localities. Poverty is clearly a major issue in Bethnal Green as well as parts of Wolverhampton. Bourke, in her study of working class communities in the first half of the century, makes the point that material hardship does not itself guarantee solidarity or encourage people to share.[21] Or, as Klein observes: 'Poor kin may help each other, poor neighbours more rarely'.[22] But in the late twentieth century, the issue is as much about widening inequality within and between localities, as about poverty in any straightforward sense. Such inequality, as Wilkinson observes, may serve to weaken social cohesion within neighbourhoods.[23] The reality may be that in many districts, neighbourly reserve may run alongside greater insecurity about the context in which neighbouring takes place.

The areas clearly varied, however, in terms of the extent to which older people reported problems with those living around them. Reflecting this, although only a minority of those surveyed said they would be happy to move (19 per cent), there were clear differences between the localities; 34 per cent of older people in Bethnal Green reported that they would be happy to move, compared with 15 per cent in Wolverhampton, and 7 per cent in Woodford. In all areas, younger elderly people (aged sixty to seventy-four) had a greater wish to move than very elderly respondents. In Bethnal Green, 40 per cent of those between sixty and seventy-four said they would be happy to move: a remarkably high figure given the length of time most of the respondents had lived in or around the area.

Having examined what people like and dislike about their areas, we turn finally to consider each area in more detail, highlighting the ways in which experiences of neighbourhoods, neighbours and neighbouring have changed since the 1950s. In the next section, we focus on our qualitative interviews with sixty-two white respondents who were aged seventy-five years and over.

Bethnal Green: a lost community?

Trying to assess the extent of change, especially as it is perceived by older people, raises considerable difficulties. Taylor *et al.*, interviewing older people in Manchester and Sheffield in the early 1990s, refer to what seemed to be a sense of nostalgia for a 'lost community' which was shared by many of the respondents. Many commented with a sense of 'sadness and even bitterness at the condition of the city in which they lived and especially that of its people'.[24] It is certainly the case that this sense of loss was conveyed by many of our respondents, both in the survey and in the qualitative interviews for our study. But responses were certainly not uniform, and varied in some respects between the areas. In any event, the issue is complicated by the fact that in Bethnal Green and Wolverhampton there has clearly been a significant change since the baseline studies, notably in respect of the link between neighbours and kin. Klein, in a review of a number of community studies, notes that:

> The frequency of neighbourly contact and the intimacy with which people know the details of each other's lives makes it easy in some ways for neighbours to be helpful to one another and thus create a feeling of solidarity. According to some commentators, there is a good deal of neighbourly help in these old traditional areas. The evidence is not very easily interpreted. We shall argue that kin living in the neighbourhood rather than unrelated neighbours are mainly responsible for what is loosely called 'neighbourliness' . . . much of the helpfulness observed in traditional communities is [in fact] specifically helpfulness between kin who live in the same neighbourhood.[25]

In this last respect, there certainly had been a change – at least for our white elderly respondents – in Bethnal Green and Wolverhampton. For those who had been born or had spent much of their lives in these areas, their experience was one of a locality where significant kin were at one time close at hand. The baseline studies by Sheldon and Townsend described patterns of 'localized kinship', where older people were either living with or in the same street as a relative of some kind. In Sheldon's 1945 sample, 59 per cent of older people lived with kin (mainly children); in Bethnal Green, the figure was 46 per cent. Fifty years later, the proportions were 21 per cent and 27 per cent respectively.

Even if this type of co-residence was in fact less a matter of choice than a reflection of the lack of alternatives given shortages of accommodation and high rates of marriage, the sense in which neighbourhoods were built around kin is an important part of the memory of older people in these areas. In our study, this seemed especially characteristic among the group of very elderly men and women in Bethnal Green. Mr Price, an eighty-seven year old widower, who we introduced in Chapter 4, has spent all his life in Bethnal Green. He recalls a childhood spent in one of the 'turnings', describing this in ways similar to Townsend's respondents:

> We were at number 34 and my Mum used to go into 12 or 14 up the road, up the turning, everyone knew everyone. There wasn't one in the turning that was aloof or didn't want to know about the others. . . . Well the other side of the street there was a little bit aloof. They weren't stuck up people but they kept themselves to themselves, they wasn't like the 'top end' as we called it.

In old age, he is now living with his son (his main carer) on the fifth floor of a large block of flats. He emphasises, in the following exchange, the importance of the link with his neighbours, though one which he feels is now less common:

Interviewer: In a situation where you were unwell, who would look after you then?

Mr Price: My son. My son, or my daughter's got me phone number around the corner or Millie or Lil [two neighbours] will phone them up because they've got the phone numbers to do that. That's the old type of neighbour, you don't get it, you wouldn't get that kind of service in the rest of the block, they are so distant to one another, why I don't know . . .

Interviewer: You think that's kind of changing?

Mr Price: Oh definitely, I mean different people are coming, I mean you might have heard it but, er, there's a saying now that you don't know who your next door neighbour is in some of these blocks and it's right; they don't bother to converse with one another . . .

Interviewer: So there is a change here?

Mr Price: Oh definitely, nothing we had in our . . . before the war like, or just after the war. I mean they were still neighbours then, every neighbour you'd see doors wide open all day. Me Mum and them used to walk in Mrs so-and-so's and have a cup of tea, and come out . . . the doors would be left open. You used to bore a hole in the middle of the door and string would come through that was tied to the lock and you'd pull that string and let yourself in.

Mr Masters (a seventy-seven year old widower) also perceived a change in Bethnal Green. In his case, he had a daughter living next door to him and seemed from the survey to have fairly extensive contacts with his neighbours. But the follow-up interview with him identified concerns about what he regarded as unwelcome changes:

Mr Masters: Look . . . nobody knows how you are getting on in your own family in this world today. Years ago . . . you . . . a lot people don't understand this. The people who lived in Bethnal Green, lived in Bethnal Green all their lives. Its like all of London. Wherever you lived, you lived there all your life. Now its altered. You see you've got so many different people here from different places. I am not talking about coloured people and all that business, I am talking about actual people who live here. They come from Stratford and all over the place, wherever they can put them.

Interviewer: So how does this affect the people who live here then?

Mr Masters: When I was a boy, you won't believe this but its true. Everybody used to leave their door open. There was no crime, very little crime among the working class.

Interviewer: Don't you share things with your neighbour next door?

Mr Masters: Well, we used to talk but we don't share things like they used to years ago. . . . Years ago it was a different world . . . everybody was the same. Everybody in the working-class was poor. These people with money don't care about you. I mean look at the blokes in those positions now. You see years ago people used to have one job and that was it, they used to stick at it. . . . You see today people don't care too much about the working class.

Mr Masters' views about change are accurate in at least one respect. Husband, for example, notes that although the East End has seen waves of foreign and immigrant settlement, Bethnal Green had for a long period a population which was predominantly London-born.[26] Young and Willmott highlight the fact that the 1951 Census showed Bethnal Green to have a higher proportion of residents born in it than virtually any other London borough (as already noted nearly one-third of our white respondents were themselves born in the area). A survey conducted for the Institute of Community Studies in 1992, found 80 per cent of the older people surveyed were London-born.

People's experience of change is rooted in day-to-day observations about and contacts with their community. At one level, as regards neighbouring, these were still often highly positive. Many of our respondents had moved into their home (in the majority of cases a flat) in the 1950s or early 1960s, often being the first group of residents. For many there was a real sense of pride in, and attachment to, where they lived (the home as the embodiment of 'a thousand memories' as Townsend expressed it). Mrs Hart, for example, is seventy-five and lives with her husband on the ninth floor of a tower block, having moved in when it was completed in 1963:

Mrs Hart: We lived with Bert's Mum for about two years, until we got a two bedroomed flat, well not a flat just two bedrooms in the house, but we didn't have any water up there. I had to carry the water up and down in the pail, so I don't think really until I moved here that's why I liked to live here, because until I moved in and had this place of my own I never sort of had any, what can you say, any comfort, you know.

Interviewer: So this flat has been very important to you?

Mrs Hart: Yes. It's been very important to me because it's been part of what I call the good side of me life yes . . . and we've been happy here, we've had a happy life, we've always gone out and about and when our son got married he went, we were left on our own, so we've always gone everywhere together and done everything together, we've never been anywhere without each other.

Mrs Hart has had the same neighbour for all the time she has been in the flat, someone who helps her now that has become the carer for her husband who has Parkinson's disease:

Mrs Hart: The only day I go shopping is on Thursday . . . I do my week's shopping. I have got a big trolley in there, and I take that and I fill it up and the lady at number 10 gets me fresh bread and milk on a Wednesday . . .

Interviewer: That's your next-door neighbour?

Mrs Hart: Yeah, that's number 10, yeah, and anything I want in-between she's always, she's got the car so she says it's no bother.

Interviewer: Is that somebody you've known for some time?

Mrs Hart:	She's lived here the same amount of time as, we've been here thirty-one years in this flat and she's been the same, she came in about a month after us when [they were built].

Mrs Foster is a widow of eighty-two, who was born in 'one of the turnings' off the Hackney Road; she has spent just one year of her life away from the area. She is now very disabled and prior to the interview had not been out of the flat for six weeks. She has one daughter who lives in Essex with whom she is very close; she also has regular contact with some of her neighbours. She talks about a couple on the same landing as her as follows:

Mrs Foster:	They go and get all my shopping for me. . . . They go and get me pension and then I give them a list and they come in. Oh they bring the paper in for me and they come in every day and see if I want any shopping.
Interviewer:	How long have you known them?
Mrs Foster:	Ever since we have been here . . . must be getting on forty years now.

Another neighbour also offers support, this being interpreted as a 'paying back' of previous help from Mrs. Foster:

Interviewer:	Is there anyone else on the landing who helps out?
Mrs Foster:	No . . . there is only a fellow two or three doors up here and every time he cooks he sends me in something. . . . I keep telling him to stop it but he says you were good to us. When we wanted money you lent it to us, so I am paying you back.
Interviewer:	Did they fall on hard times then?
Mrs Foster:	They couldn't get their cheques changed. When he worked he got a cheque and they had so many days before they could change it and they didn't have any money. So they used to come and borrow off me. I knew they were alright. She's Scottish, he's not. He used to live somewhere around here when he was a kid.

Long-term support from neighbours is, however, fairly exceptional and our interviews yielded relatively few examples of this. The neighbour's role is in fact more likely to be that of the intermediary (a role already identified by Mr Price). However, this was certainly not universal and respondents were at least as likely to mention some degree of isolation from those around them. Miss Stanford, for example, is a single person aged seventy-six, living alone in semi-sheltered accommodation. Her brother (who lives in Walthamstow) is her closest family member and they usually see each other once a week. Regarding her involvement with neighbours she says:

> I never see any of them because we have got a lift. See, when you have got a lift you don't meet people, not like where I was before. You were up and down stairs. I know the man next door but he just says 'hello' but there's no contact really.

Mr Green had moved into his block when it was completed in 1950. He talks about the estate now in terms of two extremities:

> Well you have got the extremities you see, you have still got the older people who live here, who came here from day one, and you have got the people who have been put into here since, well within the last year, two years you see, which as much I say should ought to be integrated, their standard of understanding of life in flats is not what it ought to be, I mean some of the neighbours here. I mean we are fortunate, we have got quiet neighbours, but the people next door under us next door, they are driven bananas by the family next door to us because they have got twenty youngsters in there, nobody knows what they do but they drive them bananas with their jumping up and down and stamping and that.

But the experience of conflict between neighbours is hardly new. Willmott, for example, discussed the issue in some detail in his study of Dagenham, noting in particular the problem of 'conflict between generations' on the estate.[27] Part of this he attributed to house designs and street layout, which failed to protect people against 'intrusion in one form or another'. However, another factor was the extent to which people shared similar ties:

> Strains are less likely where the old people have known the younger for some years – for instance, where the married daughter of an old neighbour has taken over her parents' tenancy – and, even less, when they are related. Old people, it is obvious, have a greater tolerance for – and more influence over – their own grandchildren

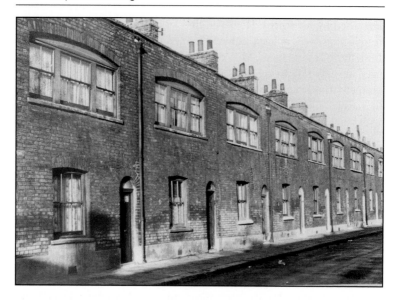

Plate 6: Weavers cottages in Bethnal Green

Note: originally built in the late 1820s and demolished around 1958 to make way for a block of flats. A man of eighty-two was recorded living in the almost deserted street, having lived in the house for some sixty-five years

Source: Tower Hamlets Local History Library and Archives.

than other people's; and it seems likely that, if their grandchildren are among those living nearby, they will feel more tolerant towards young children generally. Kinship, in other words, makes it easy for the generations to live together; its absence often makes it difficult.

This last point is crucial: kin are certainly not absent for older people in Bethnal Green. In our survey, for example, among those citing children in their network, the majority (64 per cent) had at least one child living within a four-mile radius (including those living within the same household as the older person). But invariably (for the white respondents) this tended to be just the one (married) child, with others often now dispersed around Essex and beyond. Grandchildren (now of course in their twenties and thirties) were even less likely to be in the immediate locality. Kin, if not absent, were certainly geographically dispersed. In Bethnal Green, for many of the white elderly respondents, these changes created difficulties in adapting to new neighbours. The 'old type neighbours' who were leaving or dying out were seen as representing a way of life which was clearly being replaced by something different. Again, the relative social homogeneity of older people in Bethnal Green is crucial as a factor in determining their aggressive and often racist stance to their Bangladeshi neighbours. But it is equally the case that the absence of kin for some older people added to the problems: Willmott's point about kinship helping generations to live together is almost certainly still relevant to-day; it may also be relevant in terms of helping different ethnic groups to live together as well.

Wolverhampton: ageing localities

Wolverhampton presents a more varied context in respect of patterns of neighbouring. At one level, the discussion has to be somewhat different, given that it covers a more diverse area in respect of housing styles and localities. On the other hand, the area stands out from the other two in the maintenance of what we have identified in the previous chapter as 'a local extended family' within which older people could be located. Our network data suggested that, in this type of metropolitan borough, close network members (who were mainly kin) tended to be more geographically concentrated than in the other two areas. This was confirmed in our qualitative interviews, where of the seventeen people seventy-five and over who had married and had children, the majority (thirteen) still had a child living within the town. For those in Bethnal Green, however, the dispersal of children was more noticeable: of the eighteen who had married and had children, only five had a child remaining in Bethnal Green itself.

In Wolverhampton, access to significant kin, combined with long residence in the same home, seemed to generate a different way of talking about neighbourhood ties. In Bethnal Green, as we have observed, references to 'old neighbours' were built around distinctions between 'insiders' and 'outsiders': the virtues of the 'old type of neighbour' being favourably contrasted with the perceived inadequacy of the (mainly Bangladeshi) new. Such concerns were certainly not absent in Wolverhampton, but anxieties about neighbourhood change were more diffuse and lacked the edge that seemed to be apparent in Bethnal Green. Rather, it was the loss of particular neighbours, or awareness of how particular neighbourhoods were ageing, which focused attention. Mrs Davies provides an interesting perspective on this, providing as well a reminder of the constraints on neighbouring in old age. She is now in her ninetieth year and lives on the first floor of a local authority-owned block of flats. There is no lift and as she is now fairly disabled she is virtually housebound and dependent on her son for occasional trips out. Mrs Davies has lived in the same flat for forty years, and is very aware of the changes around her:

Interviewer: Are there other older people in this block as well?
Mrs Davies: They are all pensioners, except John. He is the first house round the cul-de-sac. Him underneath, he is eighty-eight and there is a black chap, he is very nice . . . and there is an old man underneath. On the corner there is Mr Clark and I don't know who lives under him. There are five different people opposite. The [other ones] have either left or died. My friend across the road, she died last August, oh, I do miss her. . . . They all seem to be leaving me behind.

Mrs Davies reminds us here that there is in a sense in which older people can 'outlive' their neighbours: when significant neighbours die or move away, new ones may not be viewed in the same way. She returns to this theme later in the interview:

I don't see anybody only my own family. Mrs Taylor across the road, I told you she died, I used to go over there. I have been in nobody's house in this avenue [since then]. . . . I have only been in Sid's underneath once. . . . I haven't seen him since before Christmas and he only lives underneath.

Mr White also illustrates this type of experience. He is eighty-one, a widower, and has lived at his present home for forty-four years. He has no children, and his main contact is with his niece who lives just outside Wolverhampton. He describes his neighbours as follows, in response to a question about whether he would consider moving from the area:

No . . . I am quite satisfied. I don't have nothing to do with the neighbours you know. All the old neighbours have gone you see. The two ladies have died and these decided to move. I am on my own sort of thing, they are all new to me. In fact I don't know the names of them.

There is almost certainly a new dimension to neighbouring here since Sheldon's time in Wolverhampton, when older people were surrounded by children (often their own) rather than other older people. Those who have stayed in the same home for thirty, forty or more years are perhaps acutely aware of a process of demographic change (and renewal). Mrs Benn provides an illustration of this. She is seventy-five and lives with her husband in a semi-detached house in a suburb of Wolverhampton. She has strong connections with her neighbours in the street. She is aware, though, that life in the neighbourhood is beginning a process of change:

> The elderly people are dying off here gradually. You see Mr France has just had a hip operation and has gone to live with his son in Cumberland so I don't think he will ever come back. So the house-but-one next-door is now empty. And next door to that the lady is elderly. . . . She has just succumbed to a brain tumour and she has just got over that. Her husband is elderly too. . . . And of course it is only a matter of a decade and I should think the older ones will have gone. The younger ones are moving in.

Mrs Benn sees herself in an active rather than passive role in this process of change: identifying the way in which older people can help bind people into the life of the street:

> They [the new neighbours] will all know each other because we . . . I think . . . we have talked to them all and have brought everybody in. Do you know what I mean? We sort of embraced them and [a new neighbour] knows exactly about whether its Ken's [the neighbour opposite] birthday or whether Harry's Mum is in hospital.

More generally, Wolverhampton provided a clearer role of the neighbour as 'intermediary' in the lives of some of our respondents. Mrs Breen is eighty-four, and was widowed in 1971. She moved to Wolverhampton when she was fifteen and has lived in her current home (a sheltered housing scheme) for five years. She has two children (one of whom lives locally). She is fairly disabled with arthritis and is blind in her left eye; she also has angina. Mrs Breen, though, has a strong support network of friends and neighbours:

> Oh yes I have a neighbour opposite who comes most days to see if I'm alright. She doesn't, she hasn't been today because she knows Mavis [friend/domestic helper] has been you see.

Mr Barratt is aged eighty-two and lives alone, his wife currently living in a nursing home. He has lived in the same house, which he owns, for fifty-four years. He has two children: a son who lives locally and a daughter who lives in Northampton. He placed in the outer circle of his network his neighbour Ann, who is important to him for regular contact. He describes his relationship with Ann as follows, in response to a question relating to his son:

Interviewer: Does your son do anything for you?

Mr Barratt: Well, he does . . . I could go round more often than I do for meals and that kind of thing if I wanted to. She [his daughter-in-law] is a school teacher and of course except for the weekend she is really not there so to be fair, but at the week-end I go if I want. But I came to the conclusion my life had altered completely in the fact that I am, the strangeness of being here on your own, all day long, hour after hour on your own I had to get used to this. . . . It was no good. . . . My neighbour anytime I want to go round, I go round for an hour perhaps once a week a couple of hours during an evening but I can go round pretty well anytime. . . . If for some reason like I had flu in September and I hadn't been about she will knock at the door to see if I'm alright, you know what I mean?

In some cases, the social categories of neighbour and friend run together, partly reflecting differences in the way networks are constructed. Miss Barnham is aged seventy-five and lives alone in a small terraced house (rented from her cousin). She has lived in the area since she was thirty-eight. Miss Barnham actually places twenty-three people in her network, the majority of these being female friends and neighbours. Gwen is one of the most important of these, but she also happens to live closest to Miss Barnham and would certainly be classed as a neighbour as well as a friend. She and another friend were important in helping Miss Barnham after she had a fall in her house:

Miss Barnham: I fell down on the landing. . . . I turned around and missed the step coming back and fell. I hit my head on the radiator. And I bruised, very badly bruised my leg, and it was right up to the knee with a great big lump on it, and I knocked my elbow. . . . I rang my friend Joan and also my friend Gwen. And Gwen came straight round and Joan came, and went and got me some stuff for my leg and Gwen made me soup and brought me crusty bread. I mean I couldn't bear to eat it but she thought that I didn't have to do anything you see. She came and then she did some shopping for me, and then she came the next day and she rang me up. And she's golden, in fact they all are.

Interviewer: They live near do they?

Miss Barnham: Gwen lives just at the back here but Joan lives by car about five minutes. So yes I did, I had a lot of support from them.

Interviewer: How long have you known those friends? Is it since you've been living here?

Miss Barnham: Well, Gwen came after I lived here. I have known Gwen a number of years I suppose, yeah. They're long-lasting friends.

Interviewer: And are they the people that you turn to first in a situation like that. I mean what made you ring them as opposed to anyone else?

Miss Barnham: Well for one thing they're near. . . . I mean to me that's the, if you're in any trouble or if you've hurt yourself obviously its far better to ring somebody who only lives two or three minutes than to have to ring somebody who lives twenty minutes away.

Miss Barnham brings out a number of important issues here. Although she has a large network, including relatives, a group of female friends and neighbours are crucial in maintaining support. In addition, her choice of who to draw upon in this network clearly reflects the importance of a spatial dimension; with Gwen in particular, as the friend and neighbour living 'at the back' of Miss Barnham, playing a crucial role.

Not all the interviews illustrate this theme of support from neighbours. Isolation and to some degree alienation were also expressed by some. Mrs Witton is eighty-two and lives alone in a bungalow in a quiet suburb of Wolverhampton. She is a widow with one daughter with whom she has a somewhat strained relationship. She has a sister now ninety-five who lives some distance away. She lives in a small bungalow in a street which comprises a mix of houses, many being semi-detached and detached family houses. Here is how she describes her contact with neighbours:

Interviewer: Do you have good contact with neighbours?

Mrs Witton:	Not very much no, I haven't seen these neighbours. I don't see them from one year to the other, they just don't bother and I don't see this one either over this side every month. They just don't seem to want to bother with you.
Interviewer:	Is it mainly other older people around in these bungalows or is it a mixture of people, younger as well as older people?
Mrs Witton:	Well at the very top there is about a dozen houses, you know, four bedrooms.
Interviewer:	So it's families?
Mrs Witton:	The families you know. Its very rare . . . you see people walking down here. They've got all the cars you know . . . its very quiet. Sometimes I think it's very lonely as you're on your own all the while you know and you just don't know what to do . . . round [here] they keep to themselves and they just don't want to bother. . . . I suppose they don't see you because they're always in the cars.

Mrs Witton is confirming a stereotype here about ageing in suburbia: the isolated widow ignored and neglected by those around her. In reality, though, the picture is more complex. Mrs Witton's problem may be less an age and locality issue than one of social class: her background is strongly working class but her bungalow is now part of a mainly middle-class family estate. People leave the estate by their cars; she can only leave if someone offers her a lift. She contrasts her situation unfavourably with those around her, and experiences considerable isolation through this perception of being marginal to where she lives.

Woodford: growing old in suburbia

The stereotype of the unfriendly suburb was not in fact born out in the earlier study by Willmott and Young. Indeed, they found precisely the opposite: most of those interviewed thought that the people around them were friendly, and most could identify at least one friend living nearby. Although their sample of older people had experienced more difficulty making friends, younger couples seemed to have had no such problems. In the absence of an extended family, they created in fact a small circle of contacts which had similar functions to the extended kin network of the East End. The ageing of these younger couples raises interesting issues about the extent to which these networks have been maintained. In the previous chapter we noted that people seemed to have sustained active links with friends in the immediate area. These ties were certainly important in maintaining leisure and social activities, but they also played a role in providing emotional and other kinds of support in old age.

Mrs Lindsall is an eighty-one year old widow, living alone in a maisonette in a quiet cul-de-sac in South Woodford. She has two children, both living some distance from Woodford. Mrs Lindsall talked about a friend living next door to whom she provides support. This relationship – which we identified in the previous chapter – goes back to when their children were at the same school together in Woodford and Mrs Lennon moved to join her friend on the same estate:

Mrs Lindsall: Well you see the lady next door, she had a stroke about six months ago and she is very dithery on her feet. She is not allowed to go out on her own or get a bus. She has been my friend since . . . her son and my son went to [the local] school together. And she was the reason I came up here . . .

Interviewer: So she is quite dependent on you?

Mrs Lindsall: Yes, I go in there . . . well I promised her son I would go in there every day to make sure that she is alright.

Interviewer: Do you go round to see every day?

Mrs Lindsall: Yes and I get her pension for her, because I get my pension at the same Post Office.

The link with neighbours was also brought out by Mrs Hesketh, an eighty-one year old widow living with her daughter. Mrs Hesketh had moved since the first interview from her own home in another part of Woodford, following a serious illness. She had placed in one of her circles Patricia, a neighbour of her old house with whom she still keeps in touch. Mrs Hesketh emphasised the importance of her neighbours when talking about her decision about whether to move:

Interviewer: Did anybody help you with the decision to move?

Mrs Hesketh: Well no, it had to be my decision but obviously I have got three children, I had a son as well, obviously they all thought it was the best thing for me to do to sell the house. . . . I hesitated for quite a while. I didn't want to move from there because all my friends were there and I had very good neighbours and it was a very nice area, and I didn't really quite know what to do.

Further on in the interview she talks about the role her neighbours had played in her life, especially during the period when she was ill at home:

Interviewer: Were your family and neighbours providing practical support to you when you were at home?

Mrs Hesketh: Once or twice my daughters did bring me in like a ready prepared casserole, my son came round and cut the lawn for me now and again but otherwise no, I more or less coped on my own. My neighbours were good, most of them are my friends as well you know, they used to come and say 'sit still we know where everything is, we will go and make a cup of tea or coffee' you know, they wouldn't let me get up and do it. They would come and do that so from that point of view yes it was quite good.

Interviewer: I guess they used to come and chat to you. Do you miss that?

Mrs Hesketh: I do miss that a lot here because I am cut off from them. Unless they come and see me, I can only keep in touch with them on the phone and one or the other used to come in most days. Yes I do miss that and I do feel sort of cut off because it is very difficult from here, there aren't even any shops within the distance that I could walk.

Other people talked about the help they had received during a period of crisis. Mrs Hart, for example, is seventy-nine and lives alone following the death of her husband a few months prior to the second interview. She described some of the help she received in the time when he was in hospital:

> Those people at the end there who have lived here as long as we have, she as I say took us to the hospital each day and waited for us, and the last night we were there . . . and at midnight she was still waiting. . . . You see they all say, even my next door neighbours, if you want anything you only have to ask.

And Mrs Campbell received similar help from neighbours when her husband, Peter, was in hospital:

> [The] neighbour over the road . . . Wally . . . when Peter was in hospital he said to me, well he was in hospital for nearly three weeks, he said to me, 'you can come over and see me in the afternoon but

you're not to come in the evening because it's dark and you'd be driving in the dark and coming back in the dark', so Wally immediately said 'I'll take Betty over'. I mean the whole time Peter was away . . . Wally used to take me over in the evenings. I sort of think of him as Peter's friend more than mine . . . but he was there when I wanted him.

The role of friends and neighbours was especially important to single (never married) older people in Woodford. In their earlier study, Willmott and Young reported twenty-five single people in their old age sample, but with most of these sharing a home with someone else (usually a sibling). Our study had seventeen single people, but the majority (thirteen) lived alone (three lived with siblings; one with a friend). In place of co-residence, links with friends and neighbours outside the home become central for this group. Miss Talbot, for example, is seventy-eight and has lived in a bedsit in Woodford for the past eighteen years. Most of the people in her network are women friends, all roughly the same age, and many living in the local area. She describes one particular friend as follows: 'Betty is a local friend . . . [she] is only round the corner from here not far. . . . I see [her] more because she lives near.'

Betty (who is younger than Miss Talbot) is also seen as someone to whom Miss Talbot could turn for help if needed:

> I suppose she would if I needed. I did have a terrible cough over Christmas and you know that I do like to be independent, but as I couldn't go out, she asked me to go round there. . . . She has got a sick husband, she asked me to go there Boxing Day and I was afraid of going because I didn't want to infect him, because he is not a well man in any case. When I told her she was upset, so she said, 'look I will come round the next day', and she did my shopping which is very kind of her. I don't like that sort of thing but she did it.

As well as these examples of the exchange and provision of support, there were also instances where the virtue of complete independence from neighbours was stressed. Mrs Lee, an eighty-five year old living with her husband in an immaculate semi-detached house, simply dismissed the issue of neighbours with the comment: 'Not interested – neighbours no'. She expanded slightly on this later in the interview, expressing concern at the way in which the area was changing, especially with 'loads of immigrants coming in'. Mr Gimson, aged seventy-six, lives with a friend in Woodford and sees himself as a very independent person with no particular ties to neighbours: 'I feel a very uncooperative, non-supportive person, but that's how I am you see'. For him, the relative anonymity of the suburb (still in some ways 'sleeping the deep deep sleep of England') provided an appropriate environment to live in late old age.'[28]

Conclusion

What do our findings tell us about the differences between life for older people now and in the post-war period? Our results do point to different types of change since the 1950s: the ageing of neighbourhoods; the detachment of older people from local kinship structures (ethnic minorities excepted); the isolation within neigbourhoods that some expressed. If Bethnal Green was noted for its 'special atmosphere of friendliness' when visited in the late 1940s, the fact that by the 1990s, 38 per cent of older people were unable to identify anyone in their street as a friend, and 16 per cent had not talked to anyone in their street in the previous month, indicates certain types of pressures within inner city communities.[29] But such findings may indicate continuities in the way in which sociability is expressed and managed by different groups. This point is drawn out by Ross McKibbin in his study *Classes and Cultures: England 1918–1951.*[30] Drawing on the studies by Willmott and Young and others, McKibbin notes the contrast between the 'intimacy of Woodford friendships' and the 'acquaintainceships' of Bethnal Green. Informality in Woodford, he suggests, was more organised, dropping in to someone's home being the prelude to a formal meeting, perhaps afternoon tea or going on to a club of some kind (a theme drawn out in our own interviews). McKibbin contrasts this with the nature of working-class sociability. Here:

> sociability always depended upon physical proximity, either of kin, who were all around you, or of a neighbourhood with its immediate amenities and chance relationships. If you lived near kin and on top of everybody else you were likely to be sociable; if not you were unlikely to be sociable. Working-class sociability actually tended to be thin, driven by a search for privacy which in turn led to social withdrawal. . . . Withdrawal was also a result of conflict. Conflict, sometimes violent, was inherent both to working-class families and neighbourhoods; and since the origin of these conflicts

was usually social or economic, they could not easily be eliminated. Social withdrawal, therefore, was one way of avoiding, if not eliminating them.[31]

Conflict and violence is still part of the texture of many working-class neighbourhoods. In Bethnal Green there was genuine fear of the environment, particularly at night time. Street life in the urban village could no longer be viewed straightforwardly in terms of its 'capacity to divert and fascinate'. There was a 'rawness' about daily life no longer mediated by dense layers of kinship within and beyond the home. This is not to say the past offered a better experience; rather, it was substantially different: fewer older people; larger family groups. Then, the old were survivors: a nineteenth-century generation outliving their own life expectations. Now the situation is reversed: more older people; smaller family groups. But the paradox is that old patterns of sociability – for the cohort of older people in our study – have been retained. For some this consolidates lifelong advantages: older Woodfordians retained more members of their social convoy – kin and non-kin – who they could turn to in sickness and health. Old age could be constructed from a broader spread of relationships, though the better health of this group meant that it was also easier to maintain intimate relationships. In Wolverhampton, there were vestiges of a geographically proximate extended family which older people drew upon and to which they contributed. By contrast, family as well friendship seemed more fragmented and tenuous in Bethnal Green, especially for our white respondents. There was a sense of unease or (at worst) dislocation in their lives: 'Bethnal Green is a foreign country, its where they are all escaping from', as Sinclair reprised. But the means of escape for our older people (a large proportion of whom would have been happy to go) were limited. For better or for worse, this was where networks of support were constructed and maintained. The nature of the support provided in old age is the subject to which we now turn.

Chapter 6

Social support in late life
The role of family and friends

Introduction

Our study has so far confirmed the importance of family members in the social relationships of older people. Most of our respondents identified immediate family (partners, children and grandchildren) as the most significant part of their social network. We also noted the extent to which this was a more focused network than was found in the previous studies, with children and spouses central to the maintenance of social ties. On the other hand, class and community differences also still matter, as noted in the previous two chapters. This chapter takes these observations a stage further by exploring questions relating to different kinds of support for older people. The concern here is to ask not just who people count as important in their network, but whom they might *turn to* for help and advice. Can we identify evidence for the emergence of new types of relationships not identified in the baseline studies? Does the family, in the context of four decades of the Welfare State, appear rather less involved in the giving and receiving of support than was the case at the time of the original studies? These are some of the questions to be explored in this chapter, as part of our concern to examine the extent of social change affecting older people.

We examined different kinds of help which an older person might receive. Having already identified those people who were important in their lives, respondents were then asked to name those who give emotional or instrumental support, or both. Our questions on emotional support were:

Of the people you have named, which of them, if any do you:

- Confide in about things that are important to you?
- Ask advice for decisions that you have to make?

- Reassure you when you are feeling uncertain?
- Talk to when feeling upset?
- Talk to about your health?

For instrumental support, we asked:

- Who would help you with financial chores (if you needed it)?
- Who would give you financial help?
- Who would give you help with transport?

Identical questions were also asked as to whether respondents gave any of these kinds of support to people in their network. Given this list of supportive activities, then, what types of individuals were active in the lives of the older people in our study? To what extent, also, were they responsible for giving as well as receiving help from those around them?

Supporting older people

We consider first the question of the support available to the people in our study. What do our respondents tell us about this important issue? Table 6.1 sets out the findings here for all eight items of support, grouped according to the relationships most frequently cited by our respondents. A key issue from research looking at influences on physical and mental health is the value of having someone to listen to one's troubles, and available to give support in periods of emotional stress. The evidence from Table 6.1 is that most of those interviewed had someone available to provide help on at least one of the support items. The table shows that over three-quarters of the respondents nominated someone who would support them on all but one of the items, the exception being that of financial help.

If most older people have at least one person to whom they can turn, it is also clear that some relationships are more central than others. For those who are married, spouses are certainly a key group and rather more so than they might have been forty or fifty years ago (see Chapter 1). As Jamieson has argued: 'The historical shift from "the family" to "the good relationship" as the site of intimacy is the story of a growing emphasis on the couple relationship'.[1] Our research confirms this development. Indeed, the figures in Table 6.1 probably underestimate the importance of the 'couple relationship', as there may have been a tendency to take for granted that a spouse or partner

Table 6.1 Support received by older people

Support measures	At least one person	Spouse*	At least one daughter*	At least one son*	At least one other family member	At least one friend
% of older people who:						
Confide in about things that are important	93	73	69	41	34	21
Asks advice on decisions that have to be made	78	57	50	30	19	11
Reassures when feeling uncertain	87	59	65	39	32	18
Talks to when upset	80	62	54	33	26	17
Talks to about health	79	64	55	35	27	18
Would help with household chores if needed	87	62	63	38	35	19
Would give financial help if needed	68	38	48	29	27	11
Would help with transport if needed	78	35	52	33	34	19
N=	627	348	346	378	627	627

Note:
* Contingent on the potential availability of each relationship. For example, in the first row, the 73% confiding in a spouse refers only to those who are married. All respondents are assumed to have at least one other family member and one friend.

would provide particular kinds of help (for example, in relation to financial assistance).

We shall return to the issue of the support provided by couples later in the chapter. What does stand out from the results though is the significance of daughters when compared with other types of relationships. This of course is a very common finding from the literature on old age, and is confirmed in a rather striking way in Table 6.1, where daughters are a more dominant group when compared with sons and other members of the family. Nearly 70 per cent of our respondents reported confiding in daughters about issues of concern; 63 per cent said a daughter would help them with household chores if needed. These are remarkably high figures, suggesting that the emotional tie elderly parents have with daughters (clearly brought out in the baseline studies) has hardly lessened over the years. Nor, it would appear, has the somewhat detached role of sons: only 41 per cent identified a son in whom they would confide; 38 per cent indicated a son who might assist with household chores. The differences are pronounced and suggest some degree of institutionalisation in the separate roles allotted to children. Daughters appear to be of great importance to mothers, as they were in the baseline studies. Whether the dominant role of mothers (as suggested in some of the earlier studies) has also been retained is, however, another matter, and we shall consider in more detail the nature of the parent–child relationship in later chapters.

Other family members such as siblings have retained their importance, ranking similarly to sons on a number of items in the table. Those respondents who were never married mostly nominated siblings, nephews and friends as their main supporters. Approximately one-fifth of the respondents (with the exception of the areas of advice and financial help) nominated at least one friend as an actual or potential supporter. For the never-married respondents, these friends were important sources of help in the absence of a spouse or children (one in three would draw upon a friend for help with most areas of support). For those who were married, however, friends appeared to have a complementary role to partners or children.

Clearly, a very positive finding from our study concerns the extent to which most older people in these urban environments are able to draw upon informal relationships for support and advice. At the same time, there are some negative aspects of our findings. Although most people could cite a 'confidant' of some kind, it is important to note the 12 per cent of those living alone, and the 10 per cent of those aged seventy-five and over, who were unable to cite anyone in their network to whom they could turn for this type of support. There were also important differences between the localities on this item, with 11 per cent in Bethnal Green unable to list a confidant, compared with 6 per cent in Woodford, and 3 per cent in Wolverhampton (reflecting some of the issues raised in Chapter 5).

Another finding from our study concerns the concentrated nature of the support available to older people. Supportive relationships may be divided into four main categories: immediate family (comprising partners, children and grandchildren); other relatives (including siblings and cousins); friends; and 'others' (including professional carers of different kinds). Taking the total sample of 627 older people, nobody was able to draw upon all four categories. For each of the eight types of support, over two-thirds of the respondents identified only one source to whom they could turn (the average number of persons nominated on each item was 1.4). Only three of the eight areas of support reached double figures in respect of having two types of support: 17 per cent of respondents had two sources to whom they could go to when confiding; 11 per cent for when feeling uncertain; and 11 per cent for household chores. The help available to older people is, then, highly focused. In some respects there is continuity here with the baseline studies, demonstrating the significant presence of 'intimate kin' (to use Townsend's phrase) in the lives of older people. But our evidence suggests that the balance of support has shifted somewhat in comparison with the 1950s, with much revolving around the social world of couples in providing mutual care in old age.

The supportive role of partners

Findings from national surveys of married couples (of all ages) suggest that the majority would turn to their partner for help with household chores, advice or emotional support. In our study, just over half of respondents were married (55 per cent), and the majority of these (91 per cent) cited their spouse as close and important in their lives. Most married respondents (86 per cent) had remained with a partner from their first marriage, a finding that reflects the far less frequent divorce rate for this particular generation in comparison with couples below pensionable age.

As Table 6.2 indicates, older people clearly identify their partner as someone to whom they turn in times of trouble: 81 per cent of men confide in their wives, and 71 per cent would turn to them if feeling

Table 6.2 Support received from partners

Support measures	Men[1]	Women[2]
% of respondents who:		
Confide in about things that are important*	81	67
Asks advice on decisions that have to be made	56	58
Reassures when feeling uncertain	66	59
Talks to when upset*	71	55
Talks to about health*	73	56
Would help with household chores if needed	57	61
Would give financial help if needed*	31	44
Would help with transport if needed*	21	46

Notes: n=348. *p =<.05
1 Percentage of men receiving support from spouse/partner
2 Percentage of women receiving support from spouse/partner

upset. On the other hand, the figures also suggest variations in respect of gender. Older men are more likely to seek emotional support from their partners than older women (confiding in a partner, talking to a partner when upset, and talking to a partner about health matters), and women are more likely to seek practical help from men. These findings reflect the extent to which, as Duncombe and Marsden suggest, women of all ages are assigned the role of meeting the emotional needs of the household.[2] However, they also suggest that in respect of their own needs, women may seek alternatives to their partner (a daughter or female friend being the most likely confidant).

In contrast, there are no significant gender differences on the items of asking advice and seeking reassurance, where relationships would appear more 'equal' in terms of the sharing of particular personal difficulties. Similarly, approximately the same proportions of men and women would turn to their partner for help with household chores if needed. The low proportion of respondents who would give financial assistance may in part reflect the interpretation of this particular question by respondents, who may have assumed that partners were excluded. Very few men could depend upon their partners for transport, a finding that illustrates the lower proportion of women who are able to drive.

Do the gender differences between married couples that are observed in Table 6.2 apply equally to all of the three areas? Townsend's Bethnal Green study suggested that retired working-class men often felt excluded from family life, and married women were more likely to find a prominent role within the extended family. Older men from Woodford, in contrast, were seen by Willmott and Young to have more of a 'partnership' with their wives, this expressed in a greater sharing of activities and tasks around the home. Table 6.3 shows how the responses of men and women differed in the three areas. The table suggests that gender differences in support are much more common in Bethnal Green and Woodford than in Wolverhampton. The differences in Bethnal Green are especially striking, with 54 per cent of women confiding in partners, compared with 74 per cent of men; and just 40 per cent of married women listing their partner as someone they would talk to if upset, compared with 68 per cent of men who would do so. These results would suggest that gender differences within marriage have survived more strongly in Bethnal Green, with the interaction between social class and ethnicity maintaining the divisions reported in the baseline studies.

Supportive ties between parents and children

In the 1950s, Townsend saw the family as a source of 'supreme comfort and support', with the lives of individuals measured by the interplay of the different roles of child, parent and grandparent. One view of the family today would be that the bonds between children and parents are much less secure now than they were in the 1950s; that the giving and receiving of support has been displaced, or 'crowded out' as Kunemund and Rein put it, by a mature welfare state.[3] Of course, as is constantly emphasised throughout this book, these informal ties are clearly different for a host of social as well as demographic reasons. But the question is: do they still figure in the provision of support? Just as importantly: do older people see themselves as involved in reciprocal ties, returning as well as receiving support?

Table 6.4 provides information on these questions, drawing on responses about the giving and receiving of different kinds of help. Here, we take all those who have listed at least one child in their network (491 respondents), and examine the exchange of support across the generations, and across the localities. For virtually all the items, we find high levels of support being indicated, with older

Table 6.3 Support received from partners: gender and area differences

Support measures	Wolverhampton		Bethnal Green		Woodford	
	Men	Women	Men	Women	Men	Women
% of respondents who:						
Confide in about things that are important	84*	68*	74*	54*	86	74
Asks advice on decisions that have to be made	46	61	61*	42*	61	66
Reassures when feeling uncertain	60	57	63	48	76	69
Talks to when upset	66	60	68*	40*	80*	61*
Talks to about health	66	53	67*	46*	88*	66*
Would help with household chores	46	60	60	56	65	66
Would give financial help if needed	28	39	33	31	31	37
Would help with transport if needed	24	41	4*	21*	37*	69*

n=348. *p =<.05

Table 6.4 Support received from and given to at least one child (respondents with children only)

Support measures	Wolverhampton		Bethnal Green		Woodford	
% of respondents who:	Received	Given	Received	Given	Received	Given
Confide in about things that are important*	78	72	65	62	72	70
Asks advice on decisions that have to be made*	66	58	51	51	48	55
Reassures when feeling uncertain	69	76	65	69	67	80
Talks to when upset	54	74	48	63	54	66
Talks to about health	57	62	46	49	50	58
Would help with household chores if neededΨ	68	60	63	45	60	67
Would give financial help if neededΨ	62	70	60	56	55	86
Would help with transport if neededΨ	68	25	60	8	69	34

n=491
*p=<.05 for support received
Ψ=<.05 for support given

people themselves actively involved in either providing help or expressing a willingness to do so (the main exception here being help with transport). The role of older people as confidants to their children is clearly demonstrated, with around 70 per cent placing themselves in this role; one in two advise their children on decisions which they have to make. Older people are also more likely to see themselves in a situation of being able to give financial support to their children, although here the locality and class variation is significant: 86 per cent of respondents with children in Woodford say they would give help if needed, compared with 56 per cent in Bethnal Green. Giving help with transport is also strongly mediated by social class, with just 8 per cent of respondents in Bethnal Green able to do this, as compared with 34 per cent in Woodford (this reflecting the different levels of car ownership reported in Chapter 4). Both Wolverhampton and Woodford, however, reinforce the impression of more 'intact' family ties, with the maintenance of higher levels of reciprocity, when compared with Bethnal Green. We shall return to exploring why this should be the case in the conclusion to this study.

The giving and receiving of different forms of emotional support is, then, an important aspect of the family life of older people. Practical support to help older people with household chores – a significant role brought out in the baseline studies – also featured in our findings. However, there were fewer children available for this type of support than for confiding relations, this indicating the extent to which distance and commitments such as work and other ties may limit the availability of practical help. Forty-three per cent of our respondents had one or more children who would give help with household chores if needed. Almost half of these (49 per cent) had just the one child who would help them with household chores, again confirming the highly focused nature of help within the family. However, among respondents who named at least one child, there was evidence of a very high rate of recent contact: 92 per cent had last made contact with at least one child who would help them with household chores within the past week. For almost two-thirds of these respondents (64 per cent), this contact was face-to-face, and even where this was not in person, 62 per cent had seen a potential child helper in the past week. This level remained high for different socio-demographic groups, the only differences being those between men and women. Women were more likely to have had contact with a child who would help them with household chores than men (68 per cent and 57 per cent respectively). The level of contact is also reflected in the fact that for 63 per

Table 6.5 Support given by older people

Support measures	At least one person	Spouse*	At least one daughter	At least* one son	At least one other family member	At least one friend
% of older people who:						
Confide in about things that are important	82	58	70	53	37	23
Asks advice on decisions that have to be made	62	46	54	47	29	17
Reassures when feeling uncertain	81	61	74	66	45	28
Talks to when upset	81	56	72	52	41	28
Talks to about health	78	55	62	43	41	26
Would help with household chores if needed	63	49	59	51	49	27
Would give financial help if needed	68	50	72	65	50	22
Would help with transport if needed	25	25	24	22	25	15
N=	627	348	346	378	627	627

Note:
* Contingent on the potential availability of each relationship. For example, in the first row the 58% acting as a confidant to their spouse refers only to those who are married. Respondents are assumed to have at least one other family member and one friend.

cent of respondents, a child named as being able to provide help with household chores lived less than four miles away.

Finally, it is important to emphasise the point already highlighted in Table 6.4, that older people have a major role in providing a variety of forms of help and assistance within their social network. This point is illustrated in Table 6.5 where we set out findings on the kind of support given and the different people involved.

The findings confirm the role older people play in providing emotional support within their network: 82 per cent have a confiding role; 81 per cent talk to people if they feel upset about something. But older people have a practical side as well: nearly two-thirds would help with household chores, and over two-thirds would give financial help if it was needed. These figures confirm, therefore, that in most of the localities, and on most of the different types of support, older people retain ties of interdependence rather than dependence in their relationships within the family and beyond. Again, though, we note how daughters seem to stand out in giving and receiving support. Daughters provide aid of different kinds but older people give support as well: confiding, reassuring, talking to when upset; these are major aspects of the daily life of older people.

Friendship networks in old age

The baseline studies were, in the main, focused on the theme that networks in old age were shaped around what we have referred to at different times as 'an environment of kin'. But it is important to consider, as well, how this environment has begun to be re-shaped by other kinds of relationships, such as those of friendships which are carried through the life course. Friends are (as already noted in Chapter 4) an important group in the social networks of older people: 59 per cent nominated at least one friend in their circle of intimates. However, it would be inaccurate to see them as a major group of actual or potential supporters (as the tables in this chapter have already made clear). They are certainly important in the lives of older people, and they appear more strongly on some support items than others; they are more prominent in some localities than others; and they are more influential for some groups of older people. They clearly have a role (as might be anticipated) in areas such as confiding, where 21 per cent of respondents nominated a friend (a finding that confirms other sociological studies on the role of friends in providing emotional support). Friends appear to play a more significant role in middle-class than in working-class networks and, following this, appear more important in the lives of older people in Woodford than in Wolverhampton and Bethnal Green.

Table 6.6 draws out this class dimension, confirming differences on all items in respect of the presence or absence of a friend. For example, we see among non-manual groups that around one in three is involved in reciprocal exchanges with friends as confidants, while around 40 per cent have given help to friends who were upset or who needed advice on a health matter. This is much less characteristic of manual groups, among whom only 15 per cent are involved in reciprocal exchanges as a confidant, and around 20 per cent had talked to friends who were upset or who needed advice on a health issue. Friends are especially important to those without children: one third of single and childless respondents have a friend as a confidant; among the single and childless respondents in non-manual social class groups, this proportion increases to 38 per cent.

Class differences in friendship may themselves be related to our earlier findings on more segregated patterns of marriage among those

Table 6.6 The presence of at least one friend in the supportive network by social class

	Social class			
	Non-manual		Manual	
Support measures	Received	Given	Received	Given
% of respondents who:				
Confide in about things that are important*ψ	29	34	15	16
Asks advice on decisions that have to be made*ψ	13	24	10	12
Reassures when feeling uncertain*ψ	26	41	13	20
Talks to when upset*ψ	25	40	13	20
Talks to about health*ψ	24	38	14	19
Would help with household chores if needed*ψ	26	36	13	21
Would give financial help if needed*ψ	16	30	7	17
Would help with transport if needed*ψ	30	26	12	8

n=627
*p=<.05 for support received
ψp=<.05 for support given

from working-class backgrounds. Allan, for example, makes the point that the dominant pattern of marriage appears to influence both the use of the home and the organisation of sociability.[4] For this cohort of working-class respondents, non-kin relationships would have been more likely to have been confined to particular settings (such as pubs and the workplace), rather than brought back into the home. This creates a more discontinous pattern in respect of the move from work to retirement (as some of our findings in Chapter 10 will confirm), with a resulting loss of friendships. The middle-class pattern, on the other hand, of inviting friends into the home creates the basis for relationships which can be drawn upon and maintained through retirement.

These findings raise important issues for social policy: for example, that among the middle-class elderly, recognising the value of friendship may be at least as important as that of kinship. Among the working-class elderly, the relative absence of friends may indicate the cumulative effects of poverty and ill-health on social networks (lack of transport, to take one example, may exacerbate problems associated with maintaining friendships). But there is no reason to think that the desire for friendship is class-specific, and there may be a valuable role for social policy in fostering the conditions which help maintain personal relationships of different kinds.

Conclusion

The findings presented in this chapter confirm other network studies by researchers such as Wenger, and Wellman and Wortley, in highlighting the prominent role of kin in supportive ties. As the latter observe in their Canadian study :

> If kinship did not exist in theory, we would have found it anyway in practice -at least for parents, adult children, and siblings. These relationships stand out for the high percentage of network members who provide emotional aid [and] services.[5]

But we have also noted some qualifications to this statement in respect of the way social networks function. Older people may have a range of relationships to draw upon; in reality, though, relatively few of their ties will provide help in relation to household chores, transport, financial help and other services. Here, the inner circle of the immediate family is central, spouses and daughters in particular. Beyond this, support such as confiding and providing reassurance brings in other types of relationships, notably that of friends.

This finding may itself indicate something important about the nature of parent–child relationships in the late twentieth century. Wellman and Wortley note the ambivalence that surrounds this tie. Parents and children, they suggest, rarely function as friends. They argue that the high mobilisation of parents and children to provide aid for each other may work against having relaxed relationships: 'Support, yes; companionship, no!'.[6] Hence, the vital role of friends evidenced in this as well as other studies of older people.

Another important finding from our survey concerns the central part older people play within the helping network. They continue to see themselves as playing a supportive role to friends and family, notably in areas such as confiding and providing different forms of advice. More generally, what stands out in the personal relationships of older people is the marital tie (with long-term marriage of course far more signficant now than it was fifty years ago). Despite evidence for gender segregation, the partnership between wife and husband has a more pivotal role than was reported in studies such as those in Bethnal Green just after the war. As Giddens puts it:

> In the traditional family, the married couple was only one part, and often not the main part, of the family system. Ties with children and other relatives tended to be equally or even more important in the day to day conduct of social life. Today the couple, married or unmarried, is at the core of what the family is. The couple came to be at the centre of family life as the economic role of the family dwindled and love, or love plus sexual attraction, became the basis for forming marriage ties.[7]

Older people have been in the vanguard of this reshaping of family ties. Along with this, other relationships stand-out more clearly now in comparison with the 1950s. Friendships of different kinds (for middle-class women especially) have become of greater significance, and may become even more so when husbands or wives die, or where people are single or childless. This point is examined in more detail in the next chapter of this study, where we begin to investigate in more detail family and community ties in old age.

Part 3

Issues and concerns

Chapter 7

Managing support in old age

Introduction

Chapter 6 explored the various ways in which support is given to and received among older people. The findings provided substantial evidence for reciprocity between generations, but with differences between daughters and sons, between areas, and between spouses. This chapter will say something more about the process involved in the exchange of support, linking it as far as possible to broader issues concerning the family life of older people. To develop a more detailed account of the role of the family, we returned to a sample of people first interviewed in the survey, conducting a series of tape-recorded, semi-structured interviews with sixty-two white elderly people aged seventy-five and over selected from the three areas; with eighteen people drawn from a younger generation (sons, daughters, nieces or nephews); and with minority ethnic groups in Wolverhampton and Bethnal Green. This chapter reports on our findings from the first of these groups. Subsequent chapters will discuss the interviews with members of the younger generation, and the family life of the Indian and Bangladeshi older people in our study.

The semi-structured interviews were designed to provide a view of the family life of older people complementary to that of the survey. Clearly, as already demonstrated, much has changed since the baseline studies. But, through more detailed questioning of our respondents, we wanted to get a clearer sense of the type of change that had occurred, and some of the continuities that could still be identified. In the case of the white respondents, taking people aged seventy-five and over seemed to us appropriate in the sense that within this age group people are likely to face various kinds of losses and restrictions, to which the family is most likely to make a response of some kind. Our interest was in examining the nature of this response. How did people talk about the kind of support offered? How did they view changes to their independence? What role did the family take in this process? In what follows, some general themes relating to family life in old age are first discussed, drawing on questions asked in the survey stage of our study. We then consider a range of issues about the experience of support in old age, as viewed from the standpoint of the elderly person. Finally, we consider the limits to such support, with older people talking about the possibility of staying or living with daughters and sons.

Family life: past and present

Interviewing people of seventy-five and beyond provides a clear sense of generations stretching out in a vertical network, with relatively small numbers of people in each generation. In contrast with the situation in the 1950s, many of those we interviewed talked of their children now entering middle age. Some of these children were thinking about retirement or had already retired; some had experienced redundancy from their main career; others had divorced and remarried. Grandchildren were in their late teens and twenties (sometimes older), studying, settling into their first major job, or experiencing unemployment; some of those interviewed talked of the arrival of great-grandchildren.

Spelling out this generational chain is a reminder that to talk of 'family life' or 'family support' raises complex issues of different entitlements and claims to such support. In this context, we are looking at a different generational chain than was examined in the baseline studies. Townsend, for example, found many sons and daughters still living at home, a finding that partly reflected childbirth late in life for the cohort he studied. As we have seen from Chapter 5, in our study this was much less likely to be the case. The baseline studies looked at family support in the context of what were often two- and sometimes three-generation family households. Our study of support (with the exception of the Bangladeshi families) focuses much more exclusively on one-generation homes, that is, older people living alone or with their partners. All of this raises, as noted in the previous chapter, different sets of issues for the development of support. Where older people need help and assistance from a younger generation this has, as it were, to come from outside. It no longer forms part of the way in which the household or households cope and adapt as a relatively self-contained unit. Two generations on from the earlier studies, therefore, we are presented with a quite different context for family support and relationships. What were our findings on this issue from our interviews?

Family life and family rituals

Support for older people was itself embedded in a wider framework of family life, which had varying degrees of significance for those we interviewed. In this context, our research reinforces the earlier studies concerning the way in which the kinship network is sustained by rituals and ceremonies of various kinds. Townsend described these events in Bethnal Green thus:

> There were engagement parties, weddings, golden weddings, churchings, christenings, birthdays, and funerals at which varying numbers of relatives gathered. Weddings involved careful preparations and provided something to talk about for long afterwards. Sometimes 100 but more commonly between twenty and fifty relatives attended.

Evidence from our survey confirmed the continued importance of these events in the lives of older people. Overall, around a quarter (26 per cent) of the total sample had been to a wedding in the previous year; nearly half had been to another event such as a birthday party, wedding anniversary party or christening; a similar number had been to at least one funeral. The importance of these events was often referred to in the interviews for our qualitative study. Respondents would recall (often in ways similar to the baseline studies) a 'surprise' birthday party or wedding anniversary celebration attended by many of the family. Here is Mrs Nichols, a severely disabled eighty-three year old, living on the sixth floor of a block of flats in Woodford, recalling her own family celebration:

> I was sitting here looking at the television and the youngest son came and he said, 'Brian told me to say there is bingo down in the hall, will you come down?'. So I said, 'you don't have bingo in the afternoon, you have it in the evening'. I still sat here, I had got my ordinary things on, he said, 'come on Mum, I will take you down'. When I got down the whole family was there, everyone, every grandchild, I didn't know what to say. I was so choked, because the youngest son had been in the morning and he had never said a word about it.

Also in Woodford, Mr and Mrs Burton recall Mr Burton's 80th birthday party:

Interviewer: Thinking about family as a whole, do you have family get-togethers?

Mr Burton: When the occasion arises. On a birthday I had recently, and everyone of them came. And my sister's do which is in April. The whole lot's going to be there then you see. Yes we do have . . .

Mrs Burton: When it was George's eightieth, he didn't know anything about it at all. Do you know we kept it a secret. I made an enormous cake, and he said 'What's the cake?' I said 'Oh it's for Simon, it must be some do for the Scouts'. He didn't know, he didn't know until he got in the place. And there were over a hundred there we'd invited. Both sides of the family.

Mrs Carrier (in Wolverhampton) recalled the party for her husband's ninetieth birthday with similar satisfaction:

Mrs Carrier: We went to dinner at Church Stretton. Then we came back and the daughter had done a special party at night. He didn't know anything about it. It was a surprise. When we got there all the family was there. Brothers, sisters, the whole lot. All of them. Then prior to that we was in Canada the week before that [visiting their other daughter] and they took us out to the restaurant there and did another suprise party there. And so he had two ninetieth birthday parties. Champagne out and everything.

Interviewer: Whose brothers and sisters came to the party?

Mrs Carrier: Mine . . . his sister was there . . . he has only got one sister left now. I have only got two brothers left and two sisters. I have lost two brothers with cancer.

Others who were interviewed recalled a special holiday or reunion arranged by the family. Mr Barker (who was introduced in Chapter 4) lives in a flat in Bethnal Green (recently purchased for him and his wife by one of his sons). He is seventy-six and suffers from a long-term depressive illness. He finds social relationships outside his family circle somewhat difficult, rarely going outside unless in the company of his wife. When interviewed for the study he had just returned from a visit to New Zealand, where one of his five children had emigrated some years previously:

Mr Barker: I have got a son in New Zealand. We haven't seen him for eight years and he has got three children and we haven't even seen the grandchildren. So the idea was to go there. My wife and I, my daughter and her husband and my grandson and his wife, there were six of us went on this round the world tour but we dropped in at New Zealand for three weeks. . . . And they [the family] treated us to all the fares, to all the expenses, spending money, everything. . . . My daughter organised it. . . . They told us about it a year previously and I was dubious at the time because I thought it was eleven hours in the air and then another eleven hours and I got myself worked up about it, I got upset. But it was fabulous and I don't know why I worried for that year.

Interviewer: How was it seeing your son and the new family?

Mr Barker: Well it was emotional. The three grandchildren we haven't seen them. Oh yes we had a marvellous time.

Anniversary parties and gifts are ways of renewing and recognising the emotional pull of family ties. A further element (of much greater significance now than in the baseline studies) comes through the medium of photographs and videos of family celebrations. The former were of great significance to many of our respondents. Interviews would often be concluded with a discussion of some of the highlights of the collection of photographs distributed around walls and mantlepieces. In Wolverhampton, Mr Brown, a widower now ninety-two years of age, had numerous photographs recalling milestones in his work and family career. After a childhood spent in an orphanage, he spent much of his working life in the motor industry, eventually owning his own garage. The different photographs provided a potent reminder of his past, an affirmation of identity in the context of what is now a somewhat isolated late old age. Occasionally, the richness of photographs provides a poignant contrast with immediate surroundings. Mr Pinner, an eighty-one year old widower, lives on the thirteenth floor of a tower block in Bethnal Green. The flat is in a poor state of decoration with threadbare carpets. His living room though is personalised with photographs of his wife, wedding day, sons, and grandchildren. This testimony to his past is evoked as an important anchorage in the context of the difficulties and pressures in his daily life.

Despite the significance of family rituals and celebrations of various kinds, many of those interviewed (like Mrs Carrier above) recognised a sense in which the family was diminishing in size. This was especially the case with our very elderly respondents, many of whom referred to the loss of brothers and sisters, other relatives and friends. Mr Whiteman lives in Wolverhampton and is aged eighty-one. He lives alone, having been widowed in 1972. He and his wife had no children. He describes the loss of family relationships as follows:

Mr Whiteman: With me a lot of my old relations are dying off. They are getting old the same as me, see, and my sister-in-law and brother-in-law have died, see. I used to go and visit them every week, see they have gone. . . . [My brother] is like me, can't get about so much see. I sometimes speak to him on the phone you know.

Miss Lyon is seventy-six and lives alone in a privately-owned block of flats in Wolverhampton. She never married and has lived alone for the past fourteen years, having previously lived with her brother.

Interviewer: Are there occasions when your family gets together as a group?
Miss Lyon: Well not so much now. Because really as a family we are reducing. We used to be quite a fair-size family but we don't really get together, not really now. At Christmas this year there were only four of us which is the least there has ever been.

Mr Bart is aged seventy-five and lives with his wife in Woodford. He has three children (two sons and one daughter). He commented that there are fewer family 'get togethers' now but he also feels that this reflects the fact that such gatherings become less important in old age:

Interviewer: Can I ask you about family occasions, do you get together as a family?
Mr Bart: No so much now, used to but not so much now.

Interviewer:	When you say used to, how long ago was that?
Mr Bart:	Well it would go back to when my mother was alive, there were quite a few family occasions. When my mother died they slowly, we all got older and you slowly drift apart but still friendly, but apart from weddings and funerals that's the only time we seem to see each other. . . . They [family get-togethers] used to be very important but I think as you get older you sort of don't want to go to them no more, not because of any arguments or anything like that because as you get older you feel as if the . . . when it begins to get dark or the evening you don't wish to go out no more. You don't want to and I think that is the case with the brothers and sisters, you tend to stay in.

So the family remains important but for people in their eighties, nineties and beyond, it is almost certainly a group which revolves around a selective band of kin. To repeat the conclusion from Chapter 4, this group comprises 'intimate kin': sons and daughters for those with children, and (in many instances) nieces and nephews for those who are childless. It is this circle of relatives which is available for the provision of support both in emergencies and for more routine tasks. Precisely how this support is provided is the subject to which we next turn.

Managing support

As suggested elsewhere, support is provided within the context of distinctive types of family structures. In the case of Wolverhampton we have identified the maintenance, for many of those interviewed, of a 'local extended family'. Our other two areas seemed to have a more 'dispersed' family type, with older people in Bethnal Green under greater pressure from more limited resources than people in Woodford. Given this background, what can we say about the way in which support was provided in the three areas? Our information on this comes from two main types of questions in our semi-structured interviews.

First, we asked people if they could describe a specific event that had led them to require help and support of some kind within the past year. The interest here was in seeing how kin (or other people in the network) had been mobilised in response to a specific need. In many cases there had been no particular event that had required help from family members. Sometimes, however, there had been a significant change in health, or loss of a particular relationship, and the implications of such events were explored in considerable detail in the interview.

Second, we also asked questions about who people might turn to in case they needed additional help with items such as shopping and household chores. Responses to this question thus supplemented the more direct information gleaned from those who had encountered problems since our first interview one year previously.

Let us consider first of all some responses to different kinds of events and experiences reported by our respondents. Mrs Stevens is an eighty-three year old widow living in Wolverhampton. She has two children, a daughter living four to five miles away and a son living on the south coast. Janet, her daughter, she describes as her main supporter and someone whom she sees every week. A couple of years previously she had been admitted to hospital for an operation. She describes the support she received for this as follows:

> I went into Wordesley Hospital to have my leg done and when I came home I went to Janet's. I stayed there for a week until I more or less got on my feet and then I came back home.

Mr Martin was a ninety-one year old widower with two children, both of whom were living in Wolverhampton. He recalls the help his children gave him when he went into hospital, while at the same time stressing his wish to remain independent:

> When I had my hip operation ten or twelve years ago I went to Keith's. . . . I was just getting better from that, I could go out with a stick and walk around and I was with Gillian for about a month the same. She said, 'We'll come here for a month after you've finished with Keith'. And then they shared it out and I did enjoy it. But I don't want it. The trouble . . . when they've got to wait on me all the time and look after me. No, I think if I was going to be a burden on anybody I'd rather not live.

Instead of living with his children, he used the telephone as a substitute for immediate contact:

Interviewer: Do you speak on the telephone with your children?

Mr Martin: Oh yeah. I've got a care line and there's three options. I just press a button. The top button is the doctor, the next one is Gillian because she is nearer than Keith, and Keith is the third one. So I can get hold of them with the press of the button.

Interviewer: How often do you speak on the telephone with Gillian?

Mr Martin: I speak several times, at least two or three times a day, apart from the time when they ring up and say they are coming or they'll be here in half an hour or what not. I get quite a big telephone conversation going with both my children and my friends.

Mrs Burden (again in Wolverhampton), on the other hand, had rather more mixed feelings about responses she had met from her family. She was eighty-four when interviewed and had been widowed twenty-five years previously. She has a son living locally, and a daughter about fifty miles away. Mrs Burden lives in a flat in a private sheltered housing scheme. Since the first interview her eyesight had deteriorated significantly, leaving her virtually blind. She gives particular emphasis to the help she has received from long-standing friends, whom she sees as having rather more understanding than her children. Of the latter she says:

Mrs Burden: They're very kind, don't get me wrong. My son fetches me every Sunday for lunch to spend the day with them you see. My daughter I don't see very often. She has taken a full-time teaching job, but they are coming down on Sunday for the day. I mean please don't think I'm . . . I'm not criticising, they're marvellous, they're very good. My daughter rings me up every other night to see if I'm all right, you see. But of course she can't do anything. She's got two teenage boys, a husband who is quite busy.

Interviewer: We've been talking about your sight deteriorating. I wonder whether you would have liked more support than you feel you have had?

Mrs Burden: Not support, but more understanding really. I have got some support from social services who send someone every morning to get my breakfast and make my bed and wash the breakfast things.

Interviewer: So you would have liked them to be a bit more . . . ?

Mrs Burden: Understanding.

Interviewer: Of what you are going through?

Mrs Burden: They are always so. I know it's . . . I think that most elderly people find, that they're so busy. And of course my son married late in life, so he has quite a young family that are demanding . . .

Mr Cohen, on the other hand, seems to have had more positive experiences of family support, though mainly in relation to his daughter. He is aged eighty-two and his wife was admitted to a nursing home following a stroke soon after the survey interview. He has two children, a son living locally, and a daughter who lives about forty miles away. Mr Cohen emphasises the support given to him by his daughter over the past few months:

Interviewer: During this time you mentioned your daughter, was your daughter the person who supported you through this?

Mr Cohen: My daughter has supported me all the way through, everything. She has insisted on having, she paid for me to have that emergency button and all that.

Interviewer: What kind of things, what kind of support has she provided?

Mr Cohen: Oh to be quite candid, she has supported both financial and she comes up, she lives in Northamptonshire, and she comes up on average every ten days.

Interviewer: Has the fact that your wife has gone into a nursing home, has that changed your relationship with your daughter in any way?

Mr Cohen: Well I can't say that it has, I can't see that it has, I mean the only way it has changed is that she is more support-ive than she was when my wife was at home. She has been very supportive. My son he visits . . . he has come four times to visit my wife, but otherwise from that, and of course as regards, well to be truthful, I get no help at all from the daughter-in-laws or grandchildren.

For our Bethnal Green group (Bangladeshi respondents apart), the issue was coping with a more dispersed network of close relations than was the case in Wolverhampton. Mrs Hart will be recalled from earlier chapters, living with her husband in Bethnal Green. Her

situation had deteriorated since the first interview, with Mr Hart
diagnosed as having Parkinson's disease. He was now extremely ill
and required full-time care. Most of the couple's days are spent in
one of the rooms of their flat with Mr Hart lying on the sofa. For Mrs
Hart, a lady who spoke with great affection of her husband and her
marriage of over fifty years, these were difficult and testing times:

Interviewer: Is anybody coming into the house to do housework or
anything like that?

Mrs Hart: Well they asked me if I wanted homehelp or, you know,
meals on wheels but I said, 'no', while I'm able to do it,
once I find its too much 'cause I've got osteoarthritis
meself and I have problems sometimes, where I can
hardly move at all without me stick, so the problem I have
now is getting him in and out of bed. After a while his leg
is stiff and sore. I have to turn him in the night so he don't
get bedsores. . . . Yes it's a bit of a problem. When you are
younger you've got the strength to do it, but I mean I'm
seventy-five and going on seventy-six and we're just not
able to cope with all the stress it brings you. We've been
sort of shut in . . . it's a bit four-wall claustrophobic you
know, you feel you are shut in this one room.

Mr and Mrs Hart have one child (now in his fifties) who lives on the
coast in Essex. He visits when he can and phones every other day.
However, Mrs Hart commented that he had several problems that
made additional support from him unlikely:

Interviewer: How often is your son able to get here?

Mrs Hart: Well it all depends, he also has problems he's got
what's it called, it's a kind of arthritis of the spine . . .
every now and again he can't move so he can't drive, so
he has problems like that . . . and he has also just been
made redundant which has put more worry on him. He
was at British Telecom – thirty-four years he worked
there – and when he was fifty he was made redundant.
His redundancy money went mostly on his mortgage
because they had just moved into a new house so he
didn't have much of that left, so he has a little job. That
just helps out but he could have done with a few more
years to get himself clear.

Interviewer: Has he got any children?

Mrs Hart: He's got, I've got two grandsons, one's twenty-two and Philip is at a teaching college . . . at the moment they're not able to help. Mark has only just got a job after leaving school, there's no work around here you see.

Both Mr and Mrs Hart had been heavily involved in a local church and received regular visits from its members (the Pastor and his wife were listed in the network of people who were close to them). They were also in touch with a number of health professionals, especially in relation to dietary needs and to speech therapy. We also noted in Chapter 5 that there was help from the next-door neighbour for particular items of shopping. At the same time, they were clearly in need of additional help. In particular, they were frustrated about being unable to get outside the flat. They were especially keen to have a wheelchair, but were unsure who they should approach to make this request.

Mr Grainger had rather more immediate care needs at the time he was interviewed. He is an eighty-two year old widower with two sons, one living in Suffolk and the other in Canada. He was currently living in semi-sheltered accommodation. His son and daughter-in-law usually come and visit when they come to London for a football match. When the interviewer arrived Mr Grainger had just had a fall, and he had a black eye as well as an injury to his arm. As the following exchange indicates, however, he was highly resistant both to going to have his arm checked and contacting his son.

Interviewer: Since you had this fall yesterday, you haven't told anybody about it?

Mr Grainger: No, I had one just after Xmas, same arm . . . I might have fallen because I didn't have enough to eat. When you are a diabetic you need your food.

Interviewer: Is your arm still giving you pain?

Mr Grainger: Yes, a little bit. It was a hard fall mind.

Interviewer: Does you son or daughter-in-law know that you have had a fall?

Mr Grainger: No, I don't want to trouble them.

The pressures that can arise through geographical distance are illustrated by the experience of Mrs Davies, who was mentioned briefly in Chapter 5. Mrs Davies' health had worsened since the first interview and she was now housebound. Both her children (two daughters) are living in Wales. Mrs Davies has close support from a friend, Iris, who also lives a couple of streets away and who was present at the second interview. At the time of this interview, the daughters were suggesting that it would be a good idea if Mrs Davies went back to Wales:

Mrs Davies: That is the idea now, yes. They are thinking of it now, anyway. But what it is you see, my daughter has got a flat where the bedrooms are upstairs. Well I can't get up, you see. So what she is going to try and do now, this is all the talk now, she is going to try and get a lift to take me up the stairs.

Interviewer: Your daughter has been coming up here?

Mrs Davies: Yes quite a lot recently since I had this bad arthritis. I can hardly walk.

Iris: This last time it was her breathing. She [the daughter] had only gone home on the Saturday and the doctor was called on the Monday, and she was back on the Tuesday. It's a long way to come from Wales. I said to Violet, 'you will have to seriously think about going home to Hilda, that's all there is to it really'.

Interviewer: Having you been thinking about that then Mrs Davies?

Mrs Davies: Well, I have been thinking of it but my daughter has definitely decided now. I have no feeling about it now. She says, 'you're coming home. I'm not coming up again'.

Iris: You see she had already said that if anything happened to her Mum she wouldn't be buried up here, her body would go to her, so she said 'I might as well have you while you are still here'. You can understand. She [the daughter] is not a well woman herself.

In the absence of regular support from Mrs Davies's daughters, neighbours and friends have become increasingly important. Her friend Iris was placed alongside one of her daughters in the inner circle of her network, with her other daughter in the middle circle. Iris describes her involvement with Mrs Davies as follows:

Iris: Yeah, if she needs anything done, bits of shopping that her home help don't get I'll get and things like that, because she likes things off of a chicken stall, which it's more awkward for a home help to queue there unless I go to the chicken stall when I get bits and pieces for her. I get her pension every Tuesday. And we sort the money out, what has got to go here and what has got to go there.

Mrs Davies: She is my secretary.

Iris: Really she could do with twenty-four hour care now. Now that the other hip is going I think she does.

Mrs Davies: I can hardly walk see.

Iris: The only thing is she hasn't got what you would say, a good doctor. He doesn't like coming out. He wouldn't come out this last time if the district nurses hadn't have called him. She was in a state this last time and that's when I said to her 'you got to think seriously about going home to Hilda'. Because Hilda had wanted her back for quite a while now.

In this example we see a friend stepping in and providing a range of support at a time of great uncertainty for Mrs Davies. In community care terms, Iris in fact is the main carer, at least until the issue of a move to Wales is resolved. In contrast to Mrs Davies, Mr Barker, with his severe and disabling depression, has been sustained by his immediate family, most of whom, with the exception of the son in New Zealand, still live in the locality.

Mrs Barker: He still gets it in the morning. We have tears and depression and what have you . . .

Interviewer: Has the depression been something that you have had for some time?

Mr Barker: I have had it for thirteen years now.

Interviewer: Was there a particular event?

Mr Barker: No, No, I don't know. I was working and I had to retire because, I don't know, it was something that came for no reason and I went down in the dumps.

Interviewer: Depression is something you cope with as a couple. Is it something that you talk about within the family as well and get help from within the family?

Mr Barker: Well all the family understands. But I still, you see you go silent, you don't seem to want to converse with people and you are frightened to go out sort of thing.

Interviewer: You don't go out on your own?

Mr Barker: Very rarely. I can't be in this house on my own. I can't be on my own. I could go out for half an hour or an hour and come back but I can't be . . . I have a fear of being . . . although I love my home. I feel lost if I am here on my own.

For Mrs Hesketh in Woodford, who was introduced in Chapter 5, a major change since the survey interview was her decision to move in with one of her daughters. Mrs Hesketh had been managing on her own after a cancer operation, but the discovery of a secondary growth caused a major change in her situation. She describes the move to her daughter's as one of the most 'significant events of her life':

Mrs Hesketh: Towards the end of last year I just discovered that unfortunately there was a secondary growth and they said at the hospital that there was no way then that they would consider an operation . . . it would be too horrific an operation for me to undergo and they couldn't recommend any treatment either. Well obviously it was quite a shock to be told it was serious but there was nothing in any form that they could do about it, and by then I was finding it more difficult to get out of course and to do anything and the family said, you know, 'you are not going to cope with the garden', and they said the best thing you could do was to think of selling up. My daughter and son-in-law here said, 'you know we would be very happy to have you come to us', so in a panic I suppose, perhaps I didn't think it through properly I don't know, but I put the house on the market and as it happened it went very quickly . . .

Interviewer: Did anybody help you with that decision or did you make it on your own?

Mrs Hesketh: Well no it had to be really my decision but obviously I have got three children, I had a son as well, obviously they all thought it was the best thing for me to do to sell the house. When I hesitated, and I had hesitated for quite a while, I didn't want to move from here because all my friends were there and I had very good neighbours and it was a very nice area and I didn't really know quite what to do. I thought I wasn't quite ready to look for a retirement home, depending on how my cancer was going to progress really. So it was decided that I came here to my daughter, so I disposed of most of my belongings and sold the house you know.

Interviewer: It is quite a difficult thing to do isn't it?

Mrs Hesketh: Very difficult. . . . So I think you could say it was the most significant move in my life really.

Both Mrs Hesketh and Mrs Davies illustrate the complexity of decisions which can face older people. For Mrs Hesketh, her move was facilitated by the geographical closeness of her daughter who lived in a different part of Woodford. It did not, however, as we shall note later, entirely remove some of her doubts, especially concerning what she felt was her loss of independence.

Mrs Andrews was another one of our respondents who had experienced a health problem since the first interview. She is aged eighty-five and lives alone in Woodford, having been widowed in 1976 (she and her husband had been interviewed, we later discovered, in the original Woodford study). She has a married son, also living in Woodford. A few months before the interview she had been in hospital for ten days with fluid on the lung. Here she describes the support she received after coming out of hospital:

Mrs Andrews: Well, when I came out I had a fortnight to prepare to go on this holiday you see. Family is a great help there. I had to get a couple of dresses or something like that, because up to that point I wasn't sure whether I was going or not you see. And yes, family were extremely helpful, my son and daughter-in-law.

Interviewer: What did they do?

Mrs Andrews: Well my son brought me home. Well, as a matter of fact the hospital was on the way to Ilford and my son works in Ilford. He's with the Council and so he is able to pop in on his way home each night . . .

Interviewer: So is your family in a sense your first port of call for anything like that?

Mrs Andrews: Oh yes. The only port of call. The only thing deepseated. If there were anything like that you know, I've got the phone by the bed. They're always there, available.

These examples provide some insight into the way family support is mobilised. Clearly, there are differences in the way in which this support is provided, reflecting factors such as the location of relatives, people's attitudes towards receiving help (discussed later in the chapter), and the nature of relationships between older and younger generations (discussed in the next chapter). To explore some of these issues in more detail, we now consider how our respondents talked about the support they received or might need in the future, and the related issue of retaining independence in old age.

Talking about support

Many of our respondents would certainly echo the words of Mrs Andrews, as reported in the previous section, concerning the importance of the immediate family as a source of support and assistance. In Wolverhampton, Mr Jones refers to his two children as 'natural supporters'; 'they automatically support me'. In Woodford, Mr Samuels, describing the regular help he gets from his son, sees their relationship as having changed since he was widowed: 'We were never really distant, but we are closer now, since I lost the wife, they are closer to me than they were before'. He describes one aspect of the contact with his son as follows:

Interviewer: And you have a phone call from your son every day?
Mr Samuels: Every day. I had one already this morning from my son. He gets up around about 8.30 and picks up the phone. 'Hello, how are you, got anything to report?' And I have a little bit to report. For the last three or four weeks I have had no money from the attendance allowance and income support. He gets on to them and then says, 'you phone them up'. So I phoned them up and they said that they had sent me a Giro yesterday. If there is anything to do with home care, or income support, he handles it.

But the kind of support needed had changed in signficant respects since the baseline studies. One aspect reported by many of our respondents concerned the need for financial help, sometimes to sort out problems where a spouse had entered a nursing home for long-care term care; or, more generally, the need (as identified by Mr Samuels) for help with issues relating to income support and pensions. Mrs Matthews is seventy-six and lives in Wolverhampton. Born in Wales (the interview was conducted in Welsh) she now lives alone, her husband (who has Alzheimer's disease) having entered a nursing home to receive long-term care. She has three children, all of whom have left the area. The biggest problem she reported has been the heavy costs associated with her husband's nursing home fees. She talked at length about her sons and daughters having sorted out the finances with the solicitors; they have taken on the ownership of her house themselves, rather than all the money going from the house to pay for her husband's costs in the nursing home. Mr Cohen's wife, as noted previously, is also in a nursing home. He describes help from his daughter as follows:

> All the paperwork she has helped sort me out. Anything to do with my own financial banking, I suppose you see, they came, there has been a lot of talk in the paper about people in my situation which have owned their own house and so I sat and thought to myself, 'well what can be done about it, the only way is to see my solicitor'. So I made an appointment with my solicitor and my daughter came with me. . . . So the solicitor said, 'the only way you can do it is halve the house', so that is what we did . . . at least it will leave something to the [children].

Mr Whitehouse, who gets most of his support from his niece, has also begun to rely on her for advice about stocks and shares:

Interviewer:	Can you tell me if there is anything you have needed support with over the last year?
Mr Whitehouse:	No, I have been able to carry on. The only thing I find, I have got some shares see in these mergers and different things I have to get advice on.
Interviewer:	And who actually gave you that advice?
Mr Whitehouse:	My niece, we talked it over, so I tell her everything and she knows all my financial affairs and everything, my banking and everything. See, she has got to know.
Interviewer:	And has she always done this or is this recently?
Mr Whitehouse:	No it is only since I have been ill.

Mrs Thomas is eighty-seven and lives on her own in a sheltered housing scheme in Woodford. She has one daughter living 'within ten

minutes walk' and two grandchildren. Mrs Thomas (who came originally from East Ham) describes herself as 'comfortably off' and she
is able to give regular sums of money to her daughter and her
children. She reports that her grandchildren have been especially
helpful in terms of managing her savings:

> I am lucky you see. David is in the stock exchange and he under-
> stands all about shares and my income from shares. Lucy has got
> a degree in economics. So she does my tax for me because this
> is just up her street.

But in discussing support to older people, the limits to such help
should also be noted. This can be explored in a variety of ways but it
was often revealed in responses to a question about whether respondents would consider living with a relative, for example one of their
children. Responses to this question often highlighted the boundaries
which people wish to maintain between themselves and even (or
especially) close and intimate kin. Mr Pinner is a widower with four
children, all living some distance from Bethnal Green. Now eighty-
one, he is in poor health, with both diabetes and emphysema. He is in
regular contact by telephone with most of his children, and has fairly
frequent visits from a son living in Ilford. Asked whether he had ever
thought, or whether it had been suggested, that he should live with
any of his children, he replies:

> Oh, no I wouldn't want that. You see that is another thing. When
> I go away to Ireland or to Wales, well now I smoke a pipe. I like
> to smoke a pipe. But I don't like smoking in other people's
> houses because they don't smoke you see. Now when I was over
> in Ireland, it was a lovely day, he opens the door and puts the
> chair there, half in and and half out like, I can sit there and smoke
> me pipe. Lovely. When I was down in Wales, the weather was
> bad and that and most of the time I wanted to smoke my pipe. So
> I turned to Chris and said 'Chris, do you mind if I smoke my
> pipe?' 'No, go on.' You see they make too much fuss of you, they
> won't leave you to get on. I mean when I was down in Wales I
> used to get up of a morning, before them, I started to make
> meself a bit of breakfast. Then she [his daughter-in-law] would
> come down and take over. They won't let me do it. Same over in
> Ireland.

Mr Pinner's preference for living on his own comes despite acknowledgement from him of some of the pressures which this brings. The following exchange brings out this point:

Interviewer: So it is in the evenings that you feel more lonely?
Mr Pinner: Yeah, especially weekends and all.
Interviewer: What do you think about in the evenings?
Mr Pinner: Well, I generally think back over the years. The good times and the bad times. Sometimes the daughter-in-law and the son come up and they bring a couple of the grandchildren up. On a Saturday. Well they are here for a few hours. Lovely that. But then I'm on me own again.

In Woodford, Mrs Hesketh, as noted earlier, had moved in to live with one of her daughters following the diagnosis of an inoperable cancer. She now receives extensive help from this daughter as well as her other children. At the same time, Mrs Hesketh recognises the emotional limits to such care:

Mrs Hesketh: Lack of independence, yes. Or in fact the dependence on people here. That I mean is just my nature, my life. I have never been one to ask anybody to do anything, I have always either done it myself or gone without you know sort of thing . . .
Interviewer: How do you think your daughter feels about independence or lack of dependence?
Mrs Hesketh: I don't think anybody can quite realise actually because I mean she would say, 'Mum you have only got to ask', and that is the thing I don't like doing you see. So they wouldn't be aware of it really. My daughter will be the same when she reaches my age because she is independent as well.
Interviewer: I was going to ask you, how do you think your children will experience ageing when they come to your age, do you think it will be different?
Mrs Hesketh: I think my daughter will be like me. She would hate to have to be depending on anybody, but I don't think they can see that with me at the moment because they are always willing to do anything, they always have been. Their attitude would be 'Mum, you only have got to ask'. But at the moment I don't think they

understand the fact that is the last thing I want to do . . . to ask.

Mrs Hesketh's views reflect earlier experiences reported by Willmott and Young. They found the mother in Woodford nothing like what they saw as the 'dominating East End Mum'. They felt the mother's authority was much more restricted, and that if she went to live with her daughter she was likely to find herself in a rather subordinate position. Crucially, they noted that: 'Above all, her daughter matters less to the mother as long as her own husband is alive, because the older parents share so much of their lives with each other'.

Our interviews tended to confirm this pattern. It was brought out in the previous chapter where we noted the importance of spouses in Woodford in different helping activities; it was further illustrated in the qualitative interviews. Mrs Lee is eighty-five and lives with her husband in a semi-detached house in Woodford. She has two children both of whom now live away from the area:

Interviewer: Do you worry about the future at all, that you couldn't manage at all?

Mrs Lee: No, don't worry about it. Don't think about it. Going to die, I hope we both die together, there won't be any problem then. You must think about it now, mustn't you at this age?

Interviewer: Yes, I think that's important. I mean if you were here on your own, how would you manage then do you think?

Mrs Lee: There are one or two people on their own down this street, quite nice people. And they go down to their daughter's in Winchester or somewhere. And they seem to manage alright. I don't know what I would do. They [her children] would all be on to me: 'Oh you'd better come here you know'. I don't think they want me to live with them, but they might find me somewhere nearer. I don't think I want that particularly either. I don't think I would live very long afterwards anyway, but that doesn't matter.

Mrs Chapman is seventy-eight and lives with her husband in a large detached house in Woodford. As with Mrs Lee she had two daughters both of whom are now living outside the area. She again emphasised the importance of living an independent life. Asked whether hers was a close family she says: 'Well we don't live in each other's pockets but we are always available if there's something we need, that sort of . . . we're very independent people really.'

Later in the interview she talks about whether she would consider living with her children:

Interviewer: If there was ever a situation where say your daughter's sons had left home and I don't know, maybe she wasn't working or something, or where you would find yourself perhaps living together again, either you going to live with her or she coming to live with you?

Mrs Chapman: Yes you don't know if that's a . . . but it's not a good situation, I wouldn't advise it for either party really.

Interviewer: You think it's best to remain independent?

Mrs Chapman: Oh yes, however much you get on with people, its better in the long run, because you end up doing what they want you to do, and the same thing they'll have to do what you want to do, and that sort of thing.

This sense of the limits to relationships was also clear for many of those interviewed in Wolverhampton, and almost certainly reflects the steady growth of the 'companionate marriage' referred to in Chapter 1, based upon a tie of what may be fifty or more years. Mr Short is aged ninety-one and is the main carer for his eighty-nine year old wife, now housebound after a leg amputation (they had been married sixty-three years at the time of the interview). They have one son (now retired) who lives in another part of the West Midlands. Here is Mr Short responding to a question about care in the future, highlighting some of the complexities behind this issue:

Interviewer: But do you look ahead to a point when you couldn't manage, say, if you became disabled?

Mr Short: Well we would have to go into a home and pay.

Interviewer: You wouldn't for example go and stay with your son?

Mr Short: Well he certainly couldn't take the two of us. Now you see a much nearer . . . closer thing is if I suddenly fell down and broke a leg what would happen to Hilda. . . . Because she can't do anything really. Well now we were only discussing it the other night . . . er . . . I mean I don't know what you would do. You can't say to your

son by the way . . . er . . . Hilda is coming to stay with
you, get on. . . . It has got to come from him.

Mr Short also points out some of the practical difficulties which
would be involved in making even a temporary move:

Now er Hilda I mean she has a wheelchair . . . she gets out of bed
and runs around this flat like a two year old. Now if Hilda wakes
up in the night and wants to go to the bathroom she gets out of bed
. . . she gets into the bathroom in the dark and she comes back and
gets back into bed. She's not helpless. She knows this flat and so
forth. Now Mike has quite a nice three-bedroomed house you see
but their toilet is upstairs you see, and the bloomin stairs have got
no handrail on them, well she couldn't go upstairs anyway. I don't
know what if they decided they were going to have Hilda for a
month it would be quite an operation to get her in there.

Some of the possible tensions with children are also brought out by
Mrs Burden, some of whose experiences were discussed earlier in
this chapter:

Interviewer: Could you ever envisage a situation where you would
                 go and live with one of your children?
Mrs Burden: No.
Interviewer: Why is that?
Mrs Burden: They've no room either of them, no, no. Never men-
                 tioned it.
Interviewer: Is it anything that you ever think about?
Mrs Burden: I don't think I'd like it, I'd be so conscious of being a
                 sort of hindrance to them. While Peter I know hasn't
                 got a spare bedroom you see. Margaret has got a spare
                 bedroom but of course she is very much at work all day
                 and she's never, never, never mentioned it, so I feel
                 quite sure she wouldn't.
Interviewer: What would you want to do then, I mean aside from . . . ?
Mrs Burden: I think I'd quite like to be with Margaret, but I don't
                 know whether we would get on as well. You know we
                 get on very well at the moment, always have done, but
                 then she left home at eighteen you see and hasn't been
                 home since, and we always get on very well. But she
                 has never suggested anything . . .

Interviewer: But if you had a free choice would you choose to live with Margaret rather than say going into a residential home?

Mrs Burden: That's a very difficult question because I don't know whether I'd feel more uncomfortable with Margaret, because she leads a very social life and, if she let me have a bed-sitting room entirely to myself alone, but not if I was expected to join in all the family goings on because the boys are growing up and it's always full of people as you can imagine.

Mrs Burden raises another important change since the baseline studies (and most especially that of Sheldon), namely the gap between the age at which children left home and the age at which the older person was experiencing chronic illnesses of different kinds. In terms of family time, more than a generation has elapsed since Mrs Burden's daughter left home. In this period, daughters (and sons) do not became strangers; they do, however, assume different lifestyles and responsibilities, these often complicating the kind of responses which may be made to the issue of care and support.

One final point, in some cases the issue of tracing the management of care across generations was inappropriate, either because of the absence of kin or because of the continued demands from younger generations. This was a particular issue for the Bangladeshis in Bethnal Green (as will be noted in a later chapter) but it was also characteristic of a small number of other families we interviewed. One example here (also from Bethnal Green) was Mr Lane, a married man of seventy-six, who lived with his wife and two of his sons, who had both been born in Bethnal Green. The sons both had learning difficulties. Mr Lane's wife (herself in her early seventies) was the main carer. Mr Lane was in poor health with arthritis and severe bronchitis. They had two grandchildren through a third son who lived in Bethnal Green. Contact with this son had become fairly restricted after he had separated from his wife, although there was some contact with one grandchild. Mr Lane listed a brother and sister in his network, as well as a variety of in-laws, most of whom were living in Barking, Dagenham and Braintree. Mr Lane described the family as now 'having dispersed' and said there was no contact on a regular basis.

One of Mr Lane's son's is severely handicapped requiring twenty-four-hour care and attention. He is unable to walk, but drags himself along the floor and up the stairs. He needs help when both washing and toiletting. The other son living at home is partially sighted, and is in sheltered employment. No care services were going into the home at the time of the interview. For this elderly couple, their life (and the interview itself) was dominated by the pressure of care and the problem of gaining access to whatever services might be available. In this example, care and support was continuing to flow down the generations at virtually the same level of intensity as it had done at an early period of the life course, but in circumstances where the provision of care certainly involved considerable stress and tension for the elderly couple involved.

Conclusion

What continuities and changes can we observe from these interviews in contrast with the baseline studies? First, as regards continuities, the family clearly remains a major presence, notably on occasions when support is needed in times of illness, long-term care or bereavement. It is the one part of the network which can be mobilised to help make decisions about where to live, how to manage finances, or how to pick up the pieces after a spell in hospital. In this sense, the family is still doing what it did forty or fifty years ago in Bethnal Green, Wolverhampton and Woodford. But the context and the relationship between generations is different in numerous ways. As noted earlier, care and support is invariably provided within the context of independent households. Daughters and sons, nieces and nephews, engage with elderly kin after what may have been a long period of leading seperate lives. This is a different context from the one originally described by Townsend and Willmott and Young, where Mum continued to exercise a major influence throughout the life course: generations locked together (and often living together) in conflict as well as harmony.

To be sure, there were lots of examples from our own research (both in the survey and the qualitative data) of generations continuing to share much of each other's lives. But this is expressed in a different way in the 1990s than it was in the 1950s. For example, the marital tie, as we have emphasised, is much more important now than it was in Sheldon and Townsend's time. Growing old is more often experienced as being part of a couple rather than a wider family group. In particular, the sense of couples retiring and managing old age together is stronger now than it was forty years ago, and this has done much to alter the dynamics of family life in old age (Mr and

Mrs Short in Wolverhampton are a good illustration of this point, with a marriage stretching over sixty years).

There is also a sense in which family life has to be 'worked at' and 'managed', in a way which is probably more true now than it was in the 1950s. The original Woodford study, with older people (usually following bereavement) coming to live with or close to their children, was on the cusp of this change. Most families now do not live in the same household or street as their parents or grandparents. Even if living within four miles they have other families, their own family, their own working life, to contend with. Relationships with an elderly parent are managed within this context: telephones (increasingly mobile) now becoming an important link in respect of maintaining regular ties.

None of this is to say that there has been a 'deterioration' or some kind of falling away in the strength of family ties. It remains the case that if you ask people, as we did, who is important and special in their life, family ties remain the most important. For the single, as well as some other groups, friends are also vital in sustaining a reasonable quality of life. What has changed is that generational ties are viewed in different ways now than was perhaps the case in early post-war Britain. To explore this further, we now consider in more detail the links between older and younger generations as revealed by another phase of our research.

Chapter 8

Ties that bind

Relationships across the generations

Introduction

The previous two chapters examined different aspects of the nature of support in the three localities of our study. As implied in the last chapter, support is provided through particular kinds of relationships that are maintained between older and younger generations. This chapter considers the extent to which intergenerational relations have changed since the baseline studies, bringing into the discussion interviews with some of the younger relatives of our respondents. These allow us to explore in greater detail changes in the relationship between older people and daughters and sons; as well nieces and nephews. We start by examining one of the central themes in the baseline studies, namely, the dominant role of 'Mum' within the family: to what extent had this changed since the earlier studies?

'The predominance of Mum'

One of the best known findings from Townsend, as well as Young and Willmott, concerned the central position of the mother within the kinship network. Townsend reported that sons and daughters seemed to express a greater affection for their mothers than for their fathers. Accordingly: 'It was chiefly Mum they visited and Mum they supported, materially and emotionally'.[1] In Woodford, also, the importance of the mother–daughter bond was highlighted. Daughters more often lived with parents, saw more of them, and generally played a bigger part than sons in the provision of care. The bond between the two women was seen as an essential feature of kinship. As in Bethnal Green, fathers were seen 'mainly because they [were] with mothers'. At the same time, Willmott and Young noted important differences between the areas, with mothers in Woodford somewhat different to the 'dominating' East End Mum. They reported that:

> Her authority is much more restricted and, if she goes to live with her daughter, she may even find herself in a rather subordinate position. Above all, her daughter matters less to the mother as long as her own husband is alive, because the older parents share so much of their lives with each other. Here lies the big difference between the two districts. In the one, mothers and daughters are each other's constant companions and helpmates. In the other, the same bond is still there, in affection and in the care and support that daughters give their mothers – and to a lesser extent, their fathers – in their advancing years. But it is by and large less important in Woodford because the relationship of husband and wife matters more.[2]

In the years since the baseline studies, this observation (as noted in the previous chapter) has almost certainly become more relevant and is probably a characteristic of all three areas. The importance of the marital tie is reflected, first, in the growth of households occupied by older people living alone or with a partner; second, and reflecting this development, has been the growth of marriages lasting thirty, forty, fifty or more years. Both these factors have made the relationship between husband and wife rather more prominent than was the case in the earlier Bethnal Green studies. But other developments have assisted this process. The geographical dispersal of children (an important issue for white respondents in Bethnal Green) is one element. In Willmott and Young's phrase, generations are no longer living 'side by side' throughout life.[3] One consequence of this may be a reduction in contact between relatives. This was an important conclusion from the study by McGlone, Park and Roberts, comparing national data over the period 1986 to 1995.[4] They reported less frequent contact with all types of relatives over this decade, but this appeared especially true of contact with parents. They do not, in the main, attribute this to physical distance, since average journey times between relatives show only a slight increase since 1986. Instead, the key factors were seen to be changes in the role of women, for example with the increased pressure associated with full-time work. This finding consolidating the trends first identified by Willmott and Young in Woodford in the late 1950s.

Overall, then, as confirmed by our quantitative data on support, the tie between partners has become more important, at least since the Wolverhampton and Bethnal Green studies. This has certainly changed the dynamics of the relationship between sons, daughters and their older parents, and it is an issue that we review in more detail in this chapter.

Mothers and daughters in the 1990s

Turning to our study, what evidence do we have from our qualitative data on ties between mother and daughters? In Woodford, our interviews were with a cohort of women who, on the evidence of the earlier study, had broken away from the tight emotional bond with their mothers. Now in old age, how did they experience their relationships with children, and especially with their daughters? Daughters are certainly turned to for help and support, as demonstrated in Chapter 6, but has the nature of the relationship changed since that reported in the baseline studies? We have already seen, with Mrs Hesketh in Woodford, some confirmation of the threat to independence that living with daughters can pose. Living under the same roof is not, however, as many of our respondents suggest, the favoured option. Rather more characteristic, where a move is necessary, is moving into retirement housing of some kind. Mrs Thomas, for example, whose financial advice from grandchildren was mentioned in the previous chapter, moved from her house in Chigwell (where she had lived for forty years) to a sheltered housing scheme near her daughter:

Interviewer: Was it your idea to move nearer to your daughter?
Mrs Thomas: Well it was their idea first of all. Although Chigwell isn't all that far from here, I think it is about five miles, well this is much nearer. When I first came here I could walk to my daughter's house. I don't go out at all now only by car. I can't walk in the street. I'm too shaky, too wobbly. So, when I go to my daughter's on a Sunday, my son-in-law comes to pick me up and they bring me home. And sometimes . . . when the weather starts getting better again, I shall start going on a Thursday, just for tea. But . . . my daughter comes in and she phones me, we communicate with each other every morning at 9.30 a.m. And my grandchildren have grown up now, my granddaughter sometimes phones me from the office.

The move from her previous home had allowed for the possibility of more support from her daughter, while both retained their sense of independence. Mrs Thomas describes her daughter in the following way:

> I mean my daughter is very good to me but she does live her own life, you know, and I mean she is interested in flower arranging. She used to be helping at school, she wasn't a school teacher but she used to help with some of the backward children, you know that couldn't read. . . . She didn't get paid for it, it was voluntary work you know. She was a secretary for ages with the Loughton flower club, she is the kind that does things.

Mrs Thomas's daughter Pam sees their relationship as having changed since her father died, but views this in terms of both maintaining a significant degree of independence:

Pam: Well . . . she has said to me that she leant on my father when he was alive and she said now I lean on you. And I haven't found that a problem really.

Interviewer: When she says 'lean on' is that some sort of emotional support?

Pam: No, we don't show particularly strong feelings to each other. I mean I do kiss her goodbye you know when I'm leaving, you know when I leave her sort of thing, but I don't actually kiss her when she actually comes in to see us or anything like that. No, it's anything with letters that come to do with finance or any problems like practical things, she always wants help.

As with Mrs Thomas, other respondents also emphasised the sense in which daughters were juggling with different demands placed upon their time. Mrs Chapman, introduced in the previous chapter, responds to a question about the help she gives to her daughters, as follows:

> Yes, I help my younger daughter out with cooking sometimes you know, I make apple crumbles when the boys come home, that sort of thing, cakes and things like that. Obviously she's working full-time and she spares time to come up here, she's very limited really with her time. . . . My other daughter is also Captain of the Girl's Brigade Company as well, and very

interested in the Baptist Church and so her time is taken up very much.

Mrs Campbell is aged seventy-nine and lives with her husband. She has a son and a daughter, and describes herself as somewhat closer to her son: 'He's always there if we want anything to be done . . . I mean . . . and in return we're here if he wants anything'. She has rather less contact with her daughter, describing the change in the relationship in the following way:

Interviewer: You mentioned that your daughter doesn't come and visit very often; is that something that you wish would happen that she would come and see you more?

Mrs Campbell: Well I mean, 'cause I'd like to see her more often, I mean I leave it to her. I mean, she knows she's welcome whenever she comes, but as I say sometimes she doesn't get home till evening and then she's got a meal to prepare. I suppose I could say you know come, I mean, they used to, you know years ago, they used to both come here and have a meal, but I don't know perhaps I haven't made enough effort to make them come over. I mean as I say they've got their life, they're quite happy with it. I mean there's not bad feeling it's just that we don't seem to get together.

Mrs Lindsell, who was mentioned in Chapter 5, lives alone and also has a son and a daughter. Here there is a more traditional view about the allocation of responsibility:

Interviewer: Do you speak on the phone regularly with your family?
Mrs Lindsell: Oh yes, my daughter phones me every week.
Interviewer: What about your son, do you speak with him every week?
Mrs Lindsell: Well, no, he's not so good. About once a fortnight. He relies on my daughter to look after me. I think that's the idea, you see. You see I am more or less on her way home, coming this way she has only got to go through Epping to get to Harlow.

For both her children, however, she emphasises the demands now placed on their lives which inevitably moderate the extent of contact:

> I don't expect to see them too often, they have got their own lives to lead, haven't they? But I do see her once a fortnight . . . But I don't see my son nearly so much, because both he and his wife work. It makes a lot of difference.

The experience of these women reflects the changes first introduced by their own mothers as they developed new family ties in a suburban environment. Care is provided (or 'negotiated' to use Finch and Mason's term) within the context of lives which are substantially different from those described by Sheldon and Townsend. Most of these (mainly middle-class) older women would themselves have wanted the kind of independence and responsibilities taken on by their daughters. The phrase 'they have their own lives to lead' summarises this view. Undoubtedly, it was not entirely satisfactory, and underneath many of the comments of these women was a sense in which mobility brings 'costs' along with certain rewards.

The variety of pressures faced by daughters was also raised by respondents in our other two areas. Mrs Burden in Wolverhampton, for example, whom we discussed in the previous chapter, summarises her daughter's commitments in the following way:

> My daughter rings me up every other night to see if I'm alright, you see. But of course she can't do anything. She's got two teenage boys, a husband who is quite busy, an estate agent, dashing around all hours. She works hard for her Church, she's a local preacher of the Methodist Church and also she's teaching full-time so there's really, she hasn't got very much time to . . .

Mrs Stevens is aged eighty-three and lives alone. She has a daughter living locally and a son (who comes up to Wolverhampton about once a year) some distance away on the south coast. She sees her daughter regularly, but relies as much on a neighbour for support and for talking about things that concern her. Asked how she would manage in the future if she needed help with housework or cleaning in the house, she responds:

> Well I wouldn't expect Janet to come down because after all, when you've got a house yourself you have got enough to do to keep going. She does a lot of outside work as well, with different things, with different organisations, she wouldn't. So I would have to really have someone to come in, social services, to pay them.

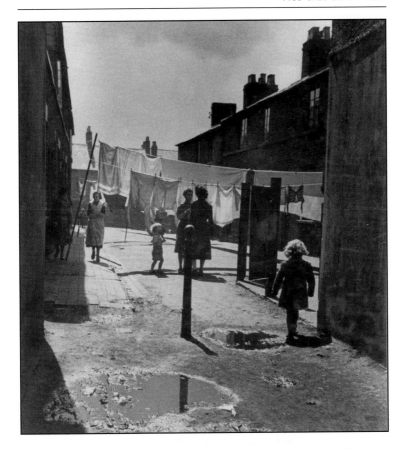

Plate 7: Washing day: King Edward's Row, Wolverhampton, 1952.

Note: This housing was demolished in the mid-1950s

Source: © M. G. Cooper, Wolverhampton Photographic Society.

Janet is herself married with a ten year old son. She describes the support that she gives her mother in the following terms:

> Well being [geographically] close I don't give her a support as such, but I'm close enough to be there whenever she rings. She's very self-sufficient at the moment. She's been in hospital a couple of times and after that she's come here for a week or so. She's also very good, she comes here when we go on holiday and babysits my cats. She comes to us over the weekend, well sort of Friday and Saturday. I don't give her any support on a regular basis, it is as and when.

Mrs Stevens' daughter describes their relationship as being 'close' but not in terms of emotional support. This aspect comes out in the following exchange which also highlights the generational gap which may also be more common now than in the baseline studies:

Interviewer: What about emotional support, do you support her emotionally? Does she confide in you?

Janet: No, no. She's not a very, this won't get back to her will it?

Interviewer: Oh no, no.

Janet: That's alright. She's not an emotional person and as such we are not that close emotionally. Obviously I see her a lot and everything, but she never has been . . . she's quite a private person. I very rarely see her get upset or cry, only when my Dad died. But no, I can never tell if she is down or up, she's very much on the level.

Interviewer: If I was to ask you to describe her to me?

Janet: Let me think. Oh dear, it's difficult. She's, well like I say she isn't a particular emotional person, she's very good in so much as she's not an interfering person at all, but from my point of view there's a forty-year age gap and I don't have a lot in common with her unfortunately. Going back to what I said earlier, she hasn't got a lot of conversation that we can find together. And being slightly hard of hearing, she doesn't pick up a lot of things people say and our conversation is very limited to mundane matters.

Mrs Franklin is aged seventy-eight and lives on her own in Bethnal Green. She has three sons and two daughters, all of whom live outside the area (mainly in different parts of Essex). She is reliant on them visiting her as she is now restricted to a wheelchair:

Interviewer: Do any of your children live around here?

Mrs Franklin: No. They are all right to me – don't worry about that. I have got good kids.

Interviewer: How often do you see your children?

Mrs Franklin How often? Frequent. If they don't come up they phone me. Thing is, I can't get down to them now because I can't get the chair in the door like, you know. Their toilet is always upstairs.

Elsewhere in the interview, however, she indicates different responses from her children:

Interviewer: Are there some people in your family that are more important than others?

Mrs Franklin: Well, John is the best. Yeah, he has got his own little business and has been a good kid to me. I don't want nothing from him. . . . He has done all this in here, has done all that for, this carpet down here, me bedroom, that's his trade. He sees me alright, oh yeah.

Interviewer: Does he phone you up?

Mrs Franklin: Oh yeah, he phones me up every night that boy. And sometimes I phone my Eileen, and it's 'oh Mum, I can't talk now, I'm too tired and I want to get to bed'. That's all I get out of her. I don't worry now. She comes up. She comes up every week but it's getting that she don't come up so much. I don't worry.

For Mrs Franklin the impact of a more dispersed network, combined with her own worsening health, has clearly influenced relationships within her immediate family. In contrast, Mrs Barker and her husband demonstrate the maintenance of vibrant family ties, bearing some comparison with those described by Townsend in the 1950s. Mrs Barker, whose husband's struggle with depression was described in the previous chapter, highlights contacts with different branches of her family as follows:

Interviewer: I mean apart from the occasions you have mentioned, do you have any particular events when the family gets together?

Mrs Barker: We do . . . we go down to the village. I lived in a little village in Cambridgeshire, that's where I was born, that's where most of my family are and when it was my sister's eightieth, all my sisters' birthdays, my brother's and our golden anniversary, we all went down to the village and the children hired the village hall and we all get together. . . . All the families get together, and at Christmas where all the children come here Christmas day. We are very close. . . . We are a close family.

In Mr and Mrs Barker's case, four out of their five children still live in London, with two daughters living in Bethnal Green itself. The eldest of the daughters describes contact with them in the following way:

Interviewer: How often do you typically see them?

Daughter: I normally go round there on a Sunday morning. My other brother goes up there with his daughter and wife, and my sister pops round. My other brother lives in Enfield, so he comes up every third Sunday or something, so once a month there is four of us there together with perhaps my children. And my brother's children come up, they are twenty and seventeen, they come up as well. So some Sunday mornings there can be like fifteen of us or something, and we meet and we chat and Mum does a bit of food sometimes and it is just a general noise, but it is nice finding out what each other's been doing in the last week or so . . . it is lovely. My husband comes, we just go up for an hour or so, and then of course I ring her a couple of times, not every day, we haven't got what I would call a mother–daughter relationship where they go shopping and things like that, I never go out shopping with them . . . very seldom.

Mrs Barker comes closest in some respects to Young and Willmott's description of the 'mother as the head and centre of the extended family, her home as its meeting place'. Typically, they found daughters much more likely to visit their mother's home than for Mum to come to them, a tradition which seems to be maintained by Mrs Baker:

Interviewer: Do you visit your children? Would you go and visit them?

Mr Barker: Well we went round this Sunday to our eldest daughter for lunch.

Mrs Barker: We go to our eldest daughter, but not very often because we don't like visiting very much. We like them to come to us. I don't like sitting in other people's houses very much when I can sit in my own. I don't see any fun in it.

Mr Barker: So they come to us.

Mrs Barker: They come to us most Sundays.

On the other hand, even in this somewhat more 'traditional' Bethnal Green family, the relationship between mother and daughter is clearly different from that described in the baseline studies. The mother is rarely the 'organiser of social life'. She may well act as 'confidant' (as suggested in Chapter 6), and indeed perform other supportive services for her children, but the relationship is far removed from the kind of matriarchal tie described in the baseline studies. Here is Mrs Baker's daughter reflecting on how her relationship with both her parents has changed over the years:

Interviewer: How much do you think your relationship with your parents changes as they grow old?

Daughter: What now? I think the biggest change is when you leave home because you are not under . . . Dad was quite strict with me, being the oldest, being a girl, he was quite strict with me. So my biggest difference was when I got married. I could then go out and stay out and do what I wanted virtually, so that was my biggest change then from kind of leaving home. I missed it like mad because it was all noisy at home with lots of children and everything, and you come and get married and it's just the two of you and it's pretty quiet. With Mum and Dad now, it is a nice easy relationship now, because we are lucky there is the two of them together. I think it would be totally different if there was just Dad on his own, or possibly Mum on her own. It would be harder if it was just Dad on his own I think because women can always find something to do. Women will do a bit of washing, bit of cleaning and all that, I think men do get a bit lost, so that time is still to come. So really they do their own thing, so we don't touch on each other, well we do touch on each other's lives, but we don't interfere with each other's lives at all.

Clearly a different kind of mother–daughter relationship has evolved here from that described in the baseline studies. Importantly, the relationship is described in the context of the parents' marriage, and elsewhere in the interview concern about 'Dad' is expressed in equal measure to feelings about 'Mum'. And despite the intense warmth and affection the daughter expresses for her relationship with her mother, the idea of 'not interfering' in each other's lives is expressed with great firmness. But before leaving this interview, to touch on another (less discussed aspect) of the mother–daughter tie, let us just report this daughter's views about the measure of concern she feels about her parents:

Interviewer: If say one of your parents died, would you see yourself taking on more of the responsibility in terms of looking after them?

Daughter: Yes, you have got to haven't you, of course you have. With [my husband's] Mum and Dad, his Mum died and left his Dad, and it is quite a stressful time actually when you have a man who hasn't been able to cope, who has not been taught to run a house, doesn't know the first thing about running a house. All of a sudden he has got bills and things and doesn't know the first thing about anything. It was for [her husband], I think, because people would ring up and say, 'look your Dad's not well', or 'I have seen your Dad out and he is upset and crying', and of course then you have got to go. It is your duty, they are your parents, it is part of the duty of being a child, I think any way. . . . I feel very sorry for some of these women whose, the kind of sixty, seventy, and their Mum's are still around and their whole life is looking after their parents, it is a very stressful time for them. But it is part of your duty, it is part of your child- hood. I haven't got a daughter, so what is going to happen I don't know.

But having a daughter is really only part of the story. Whether (or the extent to which) daughters care reflects (again, as Finch and Mason would argue) the history of the relationship, and the balance of giving and receiving over the life course. Relationships do not inevitably reach the kind of balance struck between Mr and Mrs Barker and their eldest daughter. Conflict between older mothers and daughters is rarely discussed in much detail in the research literature (studies on elder abuse being an exception). Our research is also able to say rel- atively little about this, but the fact that it is present in relationships is important to report. Mrs Witton provided one such example. Her situation has already been described in the chapter on community and neighbouring, in particular her isolation from the surrounding houses in a suburban part of Wolverhampton. She has one daughter also living in Wolverhampton who is identified as one of the four most important people in her life (she is in fact the first-named in the inner circle of her network). Mrs Witton describes her relationship with her daughter as having 'broken-down', for reasons that she cannot properly identify, when her daughter was in her teens. A sense of conflict is now deeply-rooted within the family:

Mrs Witton: She's [the daughter] sixty this year, and it doesn't matter what I've done for her she's never appreciated it. She comes twice a week, but she doesn't help me, she doesn't do anything, she won't have a cup of tea, she won't have a biscuit or nothing off me.

Interviewer: Does your daughter have any children?

Mrs Witton: Yes, she's got twin boys and a girl. The twin boys are twenty-nine this year, and her's got a daughter thirty-three. And her daughter is exactly like she is, you know, you can't do anything right for them . . .

Interviewer: So you don't have too much contact with the grand-children?

Mrs Witton: Occasionally, they come up you know, but I'm not asked up to my daughter's I'm not, I'm not one of the family. . . . I haven't been up there for two years. She just doesn't want me up and last year her husband said to her, 'Are you going to ask your Mum up for Mothering Sunday?' She said 'No', and I didn't go up, I haven't been up for two years. I just can't understand it, I just don't know what's wrong, what I've done I don't know.

Interviewer: How often does she come here?

Mrs Witton: She comes of a Saturday, and a Wednesday for about an hour and a half.

Interviewer: So she comes twice a week?

Mrs Witton: Twice a week, well she comes to get me a few things because I can't carry heavy things you see, and I've nobody else only her and she just stops for a little while and I offer her a drink, she won't have it. . . . She won't tell me anything that goes on in her family, she says 'you're not one of my family'. Can you understand it?

As a supportive relationship, this is one that appears on the surface to be highly unsatisfactory for both sides. In this instance, we only have

Mrs Witton's view to reflect upon, but she clearly feels that help from her daughter may be removed at any time:

Interviewer: Obviously you are describing a troubled situation, at the moment she is coming in and helping . . .

Mrs Witton: But anytime she could knock it off, you know, and not come at all and she wouldn't say anything to me, she'd just stop.

Interviewer: I mean, if you got to a point where you might need more help because you couldn't manage on your own, would she help you do you think?

Mrs Witton: Well I'm eighty-two next month and she turned around and told me a couple or three years back that when she was sixty she wouldn't be able to look after me, she says:'I can't look after you'. I says, look . . . I don't want you to', I says. If I can't manage on my own then I shall have to go in a home and I have booked, put my name down to go in a home in case I can't manage on my own.

In general, it might be argued that in terms of mother–daughter ties there is some convergence towards the kind of relationships described by Willmott and Young in the 1960s. Support for the old is more clearly located within a framework of equality. Certainly, daughters, even those in more traditional family structures, have created a measure of space between themselves and their elderly parents. This would seem to fit with survey findings such as those reported by McGlone and colleagues, where changes in the role of women in society and in patterns of work have forged some re-alignment in the ties between women of different generations.[5] Given this finding in relation to women, have there been changes in relation to the role of sons and their elderly parents? What suggestions can we find from our qualitative data on this issue?

The place of sons

We already know from the survey data in Chapter 6 that sons occupy a somewhat lower profile in connection with different types of support. In this sense, Qureshi's notion of a hierarchy of care is certainly reinforced by our own study.[6] On the other hand, implicit in the model is still a sense of sons being active at some level within supportive relationships, and there may clearly be a number of circumstances where they play a significant role in the lives of elderly parents. A possible change since the baseline studies is that even if it is still daughters who are most crucial in respect of informal care, there seems more evidence now of sons acting in a caring role of some kind. Mr Price, who was mentioned in the previous chapter, is one such example. He is an eighty-seven year old widower and lives in Bethnal Green. He has seven children, with a married daughter in Bethnal Green and a (divorced) son who is usually with him during the day. He describes his son in the following way:

Interviewer: You have your son here now?
Mr Price: Yeah . . . when my wife died he took it upon himself to come here.
Interviewer: Do you get any home help of any kind?
Mr Price: No . . . my boy is getting care help, he gets so much money for caring for me, it's caring, it's a new thing that's come out. . . . He's my carer. If I want anything, get anything done, he does it. What I ask him to do he does it, he even goes up Bethnal Green to get a big bag of herrings for me and all that.

This example provides a stronger sense, in comparison to the baseline studies, of the spreading out of generations: in this case Mr Price's 'boy' (now in his mid-forties) caring for him as a father in his late eighties. A further example of this is provided by Mr Martin, the ninety-one year old widower living in Wolverhampton whom we introduced in the previous chapter. Mr Martin has a son and a daughter living in the town who provide him with regular support. His son is now in his mid-fifties and he has two children still living with him who are in their twenties. The son looks back over the course of his father's life, acknowledging a number of transitions and turning points. The first of these came with the loss of his mother, some thirty years previously:

She was in hospital a bit but over the last year or so, I mean, he had her back at home. He had a nurse come in every day, even though he could barely afford it because I mean he was only on an ordinary sort of . . . you know industrial worker's wage, but you know he cared tremendously and looked after my mother until she died. I was only twenty-one, well I wasn't twenty-one,

I was twenty and my sister was eighteen at the time, and of course at that stage in many respects we didn't always appreciate what he was going through and how he could cope. But when you look back you just wonder how he coped with that situation because his wife, my mother, died of cancer which was long and difficult, and we didn't really all appreciate what was going on. We always believed that my mother was going to get better and you always live in that sort of hope, but it is obvious that my father knew that was very unlikely to happen and I guess after, when you reflect back on that, not only did he cope with that and try to minimise the difficulties for us who were still living at home. I was living at home for another four or five years and he simply sort of picked up where my mother had left off and he was mother and father to both of us really. He would get most of the meals and he would make sure the home was there, so in that sense I mean there is a very close relationship of knowing how much he put himself out to look after us and both my sister and I would be very prepared to do anything. In fact to some extent I mean we have questioned from time to time whether we have done enough but it is almost him saying you know, 'no I don't want any more I want to maintain my independence'.

His son moved away from the area for a period and returned with thoughts about what should be done for his father:

We have wondered for some time, I mean he has lived on his own for some thirty-odd odd years now, when my mother died which is thirty-two years ago. We have worked away from Wolverhampton, I mean when we came back twenty years ago you start to think you know, should you provide a home for him, should you buy a house that is big enough, should you have a 'granny flat' or something like that? But we found that even at Christmas when we would say, 'right, come and stay with us for a week', you know, after two days he wants to get back. 'Oh, I need to go back, I need to check that everything is alright, that the pipes are working, that there is this, that and the other.'

In late old age, however, the wheel of dependency has begun to turn full circle. Thirty years on from when the father was 'ensuring the home was there', the support is returned:

Well I mean, it has changed as he has got older and now we, I mean, we used to visit him every Sunday and we would always have tea with him and the boys would come along, and that would be the main sort of cornerstone of regular contact. As he has got older, what happens now is he comes to lunch with us on a Sunday, so every Sunday he is picked up, one of the lads normally goes over and picks him up, and he comes and has lunch with us and stays for the afternoon and about tea time he always asks to get back and we take him back. That's our main contact other than telephone calls or other events, if there are problems I will pop over there. That's the cornerstone for me and again, I am not sure if you have picked up from interviews with my father, but my sister will go over every Thursday afternoon and take him to the post office to get his pension and take him shopping and whatever he needs. So she will go over on a Thursday afternoon, and so in between those two sort of key events of the week we simply phone or respond, or call in if we think there is a problem or he needs additional help, but that's the way that we have got into a routine.

The problem (and the gains) which may be attached to this 'stretching' of generations is further illustrated in the case of Mrs Davies. She lives in an upstairs council-owned flat and is now in her nineti-eth year. She has one son (a daughter died some years previously) who also lives in Wolverhampton. Her son is now in his early sixties and took early retirement after being diagnosed as having a serious heart problem. He is married with two children, both of whom are living away from the area. Just prior to the interview with the son they had experienced major crises at both ends of the generational spectrum:

Interviewer: Mrs Davies has been in hospital I gather since I inter-viewed her?

Mr Davies: Well what happened briefly. My wife's mother was in a nursing home, we got a phone call at midnight one night. . . . We went out and took care of her most of the night. The next day we returned she wasn't any better. . . . She was worse in fact. Basically she was taken to hospital but died before being admitted. We had arranged to go down to Oxford to collect our daughter and her two children, and we got back here and I rushed off to Mum's to tell her the bad news about my mother-in-law and found that she'd been lying on the deck for a couple of days. . . . She'd got hypothermia, a couple of damp patches on her back, she'd got some friction burns dragging herself along.

Mrs Davies was admitted to hospital for six weeks during which time her son was also hospitalised for five days with a return of his heart problem. One of his grandchildren was also taken ill during this period and had to receive emergency care. The interview with Mr Davies conveyed the vivid impression of a crisis affecting three different generations, and the difficulties of coping with the associated pressures.

A number of our interviews highlighted the role of sons in the context of different types of family crisis. An example here is provided by Mr Jones who is seventy-eight and lives on a large council estate in Wolverhampton. Mr Jones is married but has lived alone since 1990 when his wife was admitted to a nearby nursing home, following her gradual deterioration as result of multi-infarct dementia. They have been married for fifty-five years. Hilda, his wife, appears in the inner circle of his network along with his son and daughter, both of whom live in Wolverhampton. Mr Jones has five grandchildren, mainly teenagers still at school. His son works as a night-care assistant in a residential home in the area, and is therefore 'available' for his children, whom he collects from school, and for visiting and helping his father. The family is described by Mr Jones as extremely important and he comments that they are 'little islands of solidity and value among chaos'. His attempts to support his wife at home succeeded until he was forced to enter hospital for a heart operation and had to call for support from his family. Crossing the boundary of the relationship to accept help only came after a crisis:

I didn't call for support; John and Edwina [his daughter] knew that Hilda wasn't quite the same as she had been and I didn't go into details . . . I didn't bother them. So when I had to go into hospital myself I talked it over with this chap, they then had to look after Hilda as best they could which was pretty awkward. I think Edwina settled to have her weekends full-time and John looked after her during the day . . . the best he could. It was then that I found out what was really going on. I then had lots of support; I was inundated with a wealth of visitors and do-gooders and over-eighty-five visits, whoever that was, for some time. I got meals-on-wheels knocking at the door, cleaning and doing all the work for me, that's when I came out of hospital.

The immediate family provided a variety of support as well as calling upon formal services. In reflecting on the help provided, Mr Jones's son John talks of the difficulty of 'working through' with his father the kind of help which was needed:

So there was a degree of coming in and giving a little break as much as anything else, taking over, looking after Mum for a time, letting him go out on an evening, covering for him you know various times when he had to go out or went out and Mum started going into a panic; so mainly the support was for my Mum more so than my Dad, obviously helping him during the very difficult time when Mum was getting too difficult for Dad to look after. He wouldn't accept my full support at that point, because obviously I could have looked after Mum with ease, but with Dad there it was a virtual impossibility. It was a very diffi- cult time that was for us. There obviously were physical help and emotional help, and trying to get my dad to realise when he couldn't cope any more it was a very difficult point.

Mr Jones visits his son and tends to confide in him more than anyone else. The close relationship between father and son is reflected in both of the interviews. He comments: 'These kids of mine, they don't do it out of duty it's obvious they don't, they do it because they love me and that's it'. Similarly:

John: I suppose from both sides it's a father caring for a son on his side, cause I mean he does a good job of that and on my side I try to do what I can for my dad and also obviously there's a lot of love for my dad, which seems to mask some of the things that go on. You don't see the situations as quite as they really are because you care so much and I've always been fairly close to my dad, on my side, whatever he said on that. . . . We've always been very close but obviously in the last year it's been sort of me giving out more as time goes on. I expect that to be a natural rule of thumb, 'cause that's the way you should work. Unfortunately society today doesn't necessarily allow that to work so I'm doing my best to make sure I can, I have had to work as far as possible. So I try to be a good son in the sense of what a son should be, but I don't know if I'll succeed or not, I'm not the judge, I'm not the judge on that. Yeah, as I say, you're talking emotions there and I've got a lot of love for dad. I might sound critical sometimes but I'm not actually in real terms. I care a lot for dad and because I care I'm like the way I am.

Interviewer: Does he give you yourself any emotional support, would you say?

John: Yes at times definitely. Particularly if the kids are sending me up the wall, I can come down here and talk it over with dad and calm myself down, that you know it's quite a major thing – emotional support at times – I suppose that can be . . . yes.

Finally, the tie between sons and parents may itself be changed by particular events. The experience of divorce is one example which has become more common since the baseline studies. Mrs Campbell's attachment to her son has already been noted. She talked about this in some detail in the interview discussing a time in which they had lent him some money:

Interviewer: If the same situation arose in relation to your daughter would you lend her money as well, or would you just lend to Peter?

Mrs Campbell: I'd think about it (laughs) yes. I mean. Peter was, has done things for us, if you know what I mean.

Interviewer: What kind of things?

Mrs Campbell: Well . . . just sort of little things. For instance we have got a . . . tree outside and our next-door neighbour cut it right down for us and we were talking on the phone and Peter was coming over the following day I think and he was saying about this and he said, 'well don't worry about getting the stuff down to the tip', he said. 'I'll bring the trailer over', and I mean he took it all away. It would have been three or four trips for us to go down to the rubbish tip.

Interviewer: So practical things like that?

Mrs Campbell: Oh yes.

Interviewer:	Could you ring him up and call on him to do these kind of things, or would you wait for him to ask?
Mrs Campbell:	Oh yes you could ask him to do anything. I mean I dare say if I asked my daughter she would, but I wouldn't ask her.
Interviewer:	It's a different kind of relationship?
Mrs Campbell:	Yes, I mean as I say when we meet we are on the best of terms but . . . there are a lot of gaps between seeing each other.

Mrs Campbell's son acknowledges both the help he gives his parents and the support that he receives. He talks about this in the following way:

> Yes, they are always there for me, I haven't needed them much over the last few years. He [his Dad] gave me some money when I bought the property in Suffolk – it was a loan. Then last year we went to France for the day and on the trip he said totally forget the loan. But he's always been there for me, through from when I started [his business] right at the start. . . . He lent me the money for that. . . . I think we are always there for each other and if we want anything either of us, we'll ask and it's handled that's all.

In his own case, he feels that the support he receives has increased since the divorce:

Interviewer:	When you talked about receiving support from them, financial support, is that something that's continued all through your life or is this different that's happened recently?
Peter:	Because it's increased since my divorce. With the divorce and the settlement of the divorce, that my wife took the house and virtually the contents and that's left the business. But it left me, it would have left me homeless had I not moved in with someone else. And that's one of reasons that he was supportive at that time. They wanted me to move back home at one time.

These examples demonstrate the different aspects of the ties between parents and children in our survey. Important though these are, however, other types of relationships may be important to older people, especially among those childless or widowed. The next section considers this issue in more detail, focusing on the nieces and nephews of those interviewed in the qualitative part of our study.

The role of nieces and nephews

Earlier chapters have already commented on the importance of nieces and nephews for some elderly people. Our qualitative interviews included a number with people who identified either a niece or a nephew as significant in their network, and in some cases we have interviews with the key person identified. What do these interviews tell us about the characteristics of this relationship?

Mrs Leeson is seventy-eight and is a single woman who lives in a flat in a tower block in Bethnal Green. She has a small personal network which lists just four people: two nephews, a niece and a cousin. She comes from a Jewish family and she describes the early part of her life as follows:

> I lived at home with my father and mother and brother from birth till the war broke out and then I was evacuated. I was working for the Ministry of Food and then the Department was evacuated to Colwyn Bay in North Wales. My mother, father and brother came down there. My father was very ill and they lived in Colwyn Bay just for a few months, and then the three of them came back from London and my father died in hospital. And then some years later my mother and I came back to Bethnal Green and we lived together until she died in 1956.

Mrs Leeson remained living in her mother's house until it was claimed by re-development and she was moved to the first floor of her new accommodation in the early 1970s. Her niece and nephews were her brother's children and she had been fairly involved with them when young: 'When they were smaller and younger and my brother was living in Bethnal Green in the next street, I would often take the children out at weekends and so we were close at that stage of their lives.'

Her brother died three years ago and most of her contact now is with the youngest nephew (now in his thirties with his own family) who lives in Wembley. The older nephew and the niece live further out in Essex and along the south coast. Mrs Leeson is in regular contact (mainly over the phone) with her younger nephew whom she describes as someone who 'rings to tell me about his troubles'. She also provides help with money when he 'gets into a bit of trouble financially'. The interview with the nephew confirmed this financial support. He commented on his regular calls over the phone, saying that: 'I speak to her about her depression and I talk to her a bit . . . so I try and help her as much as I can'. In relation to the financial support, he places this both in a general family context, as well as reflecting problems of his own:

> She's only herself to look after and she's saved a lot of money. She's helped me out you know and given me loans and I haven't paid her back. She's helped me out at the moment with my car insurance which I was supposed to have paid last month. But she has lent me money they way she used to lend money to my father. She taught me as a child and also I was quite behind, I wasn't dyslexic not as bad as that, but I was behind. She used to teach me arithmetic basically, English, well basic English and stuff like that. So she was supportive in a funny way. She loved her funny ways, but we've all got funny ways.

Miss Lyon is also single, living alone in a three-storey block of flats in Wolverhampton. She is now in her mid-seventies and has strong links with different members of her family, notably two nieces. One of these, also single, lives some distance away, but Miss Lyon still sees her regularly and the two go away together for holidays. The other niece, who is married with three children, lives around seven miles away and she describes their contact as follows:

> And as I say, I think its a relatively close family. I think it has happened normally as you get married and have your children, obviously you have to spread yourself around a little bit more, you know, as you do. But since Mum died, I used to go and see Mum every Saturday you see. And when Mum died it makes you realise how few people of your immediate side of the family you have left. And Auntie Marg started to come over here every Saturday, didn't she? Then we might go to the theatre, we go to the ballet, whatever if there is something on we go to that. Other than that its just a social afternoon really.

Further into the interview she reflects on the way in which her relationship with her Auntie changed with the death of her mother:

Interviewer:	Has her (Miss Lyon) growing older changed your relationship very much?
Niece:	I suppose in one way, yes, I suppose in one way she has become my mother.
Niece's husband:	I think you needed her more than she needed you, after your mother died.
Niece:	Yes, I think so. And she was there. It took me four years to get over Mum's death. It hit me very badly and I did not cope well did. . . . Then I still needed somebody else, and Auntie Marg was there. And yes, I think I look on her as my Mum really, you know someone to be there really.

One practical outcome of this was the arrangement of regular visits around the time in the week that Mrs Lyon's niece visited her own mother:

> I talked to her about seeing her on Saturday like I used to see Mum. She has very pleased about that because she was worried that without Mum I would lose contact with her, and she did actually say that. So it was . . . it was six of one and half a dozen of the other.

Mr Hazel, also in Wolverhampton, was another of our respondents who had listed a niece as an important contact (one of four people in his inner circle). Mr Hazel was born in Ireland and had spent most of his life working as a pub licensee. He has one son (his only child) living in Kidderminster, around seventeen miles away, whom he sees most Saturdays. Mr Hazel's wife died three years ago. He has been in his present home, a bungalow, for a period of twelve months. His niece, Mrs Davis, whose parents were also Irish, also lives in Wolverhampton and is more immediately available to provide help if needed. Asked to describe her relationship with him she responds:

> We get on really well. He is a lovely man and he is full of stories about the old days in Ireland. I could listen to him forever. He is very easy, he's witty, he's funny. Even my children, sort of, will go and have a drink with him, you know; my sons can sit and talk to him. So he's a very easy sort of man.

Mrs Davis speaks to him on the phone at least once a week, and will usually see him at least once a fortnight. Asked if she would provide shopping and other sorts of help if he were ill, she responds:

Niece: I'm fairly certain yes. Again his daughter-in-law you see lives too far away and her children are a lot smaller than mine, so she wouldn't be able to do that. So yes it would be me.

Interviewer: What happens if he had a serious illness, do you think that would . . .

Niece: Depending on what it was [pause] I could do, I would do, a daily I think definitely. I feel it should be me, you know. What it would entail then I don't know, it would depend . . .

Interviewer: I mean do you foresee a possibility that if Mr Hazel had a particularly serious problem that he would come and stay here or is that pushing it too far in terms of what . . .

Niece: I've thought about that, because my husband's father doesn't live far away and he's on his own, so it's a very similar thing and I really don't know what I would do, because they are all at home, mine [her children] are all at home. We've got three bedrooms and they're all full. So then I don't know how I would handle that.

As well as providing any immediate help that was needed in emergency, Mrs Davis also saw herself and her family providing financial help to Mr Hazel. They go twice a year to visit relatives in Ireland, often taking Mr Hazel and paying for his airline ticket. They also make sure he is able to keep up his social interests:

> I know he loves to go out for a drink and I am glad he does, because again it's company and he keeps in touch with different fellows he meets in town, and I mean for one present we gave him last year was £30 worth of taxi fares over Christmas so he could go backwards and forwards to have a drink.

Giving financial support and reassurance is thus seen as an important part of what Mrs Davis feels able to do for her uncle:

> We don't really go into detail about money, I just know from little things that he hadn't got. . . . That's why we try and do little bits, like taking him with us if we are going to Ireland. He had a new

gas bill and he, we were on the phone and he was very worried about it and it was the first bill I think from [his new house]. Well it was a smaller place and he's very careful about the heating and it was £150. . . . So I said, 'well don't do anything until you get them to come down and check your meter, it might be leaking' I said, 'or it might be wrong'. Well it turned out just to be an estimate and he paid much less in the end. So that was one crisis over. But I think that is one of my biggest regrets: money, that they haven't got more money. I'd love to see him being able to do and go on lots of different things, although he's comfortable, you know, he doesn't go without, I don't think that.

Conclusion

This chapter has viewed the management of support from the standpoint of different generations. The findings reinforce earlier observations about changes in the way in which relationships are managed, with a clear emphasis on the importance of maintaining independence in late old age. Our interviews demonstrate the different way in which relationships are negotiated now in contrast with the baseline studies, with a 'dominant Mum' being replaced by more equal relationships between children and parents. Of equal significance, though, is the way in which the 'stretching of generations' creates pressures on middle as well as older generations (as the example of Mrs Davies' son makes clear). Again, this is a substantial change from the earlier studies which typically described relationships between older people and children at much younger ages (often still living at home). Our interviews show elderly parents working out how best to respond to children who may themselves be undergoing stresses associated with illnesses in middle age, or the experience of retirement. The way in which old age is constructed through different generational experiences is almost certainly stronger now than at the time of the baseline studies. Moreover, it is especially strong among certain groups of older people. To illustrate this point, we now turn to our interviews with minority ethnic groups in Bethnal Green and Wolverhampton.

Chapter 9

Family care and support in ethnic minority groups

Introduction

This chapter examines some of the issues facing older people in the main ethnic groups in two of our areas: Bengalis in Bethnal Green and Indians in Wolverhampton. The main focus is on information gathered in the second phase of our study. Given that changes in ethnic composition have been highly significant for two of our three areas, we were interested in collecting data about the impact of this on family structure and family support. To this end, we undertook a series of in-depth interviews with a sub-sample from the main minority ethnic groups, using interpreters and community workers in the two areas. This was complemented with information collected through focus groups. This chapter reports on our findings, beginning with the group of older men and women originally from Bangladesh, who were interviewed in our Bethnal Green sample.

Bangladeshis in Britain: the national picture

Bengali respondents comprised a small but an important group of those surveyed in Bethnal Green. Data on the characteristics of Bangladeshis is available both through census data, and the National Survey of Ethnic Minorities.[1] The 1991 Census confirmed that Bangladeshis have a number of characteristics which make them distinctive from other ethnic minority groups. The first of these is that they are predominantly a young population. The 1991 Census recorded 163,000 Bangladeshis, just under half of whom were under the age of sixteen, and around three quarters of whom were under thirty-five. Of the total population, just 2,000 were sixty-five and over. The National Survey of Ethnic Minorities (NSEM) carried out in 1994, found 48 per cent of the Bangladeshi respondents under fifteen; 48 per cent between sixteen and fifty-nine, and 4 per cent over sixty. [2]

The Bangladeshis are also distinctive in the high proportion of males within the population, with census data showing 10 per cent more males than females. One reason for this is the different migration history of the Bangladeshis, with the characteristic pattern of men migrating first and only joined by their wives much later. This is a feature of South Asian migration in general but it is particularly noticeable among the Bangladeshis, who are the more recent migrants, and who have been the slowest to complete the migration of whole families. In line with this, the NSEM found that three out of ten Bangladeshi adults (mostly women and adult offspring) had arrived in Britain since the mid-1980s.

A third important characteristic concerns both the geographical clustering of the Bangladeshis, and the nature of their accommodation. Inner London is home to 41 per cent of all Bangladeshis, with Tower Hamlets taking the largest proportion. Regarding housing, 35 per cent of Bangladeshis are council tenants, and 37 per cent live in flats or bed-sits. Bangladeshis are also more likely to live in accommodation more than three storeys high: nearly six out of ten did so according to the

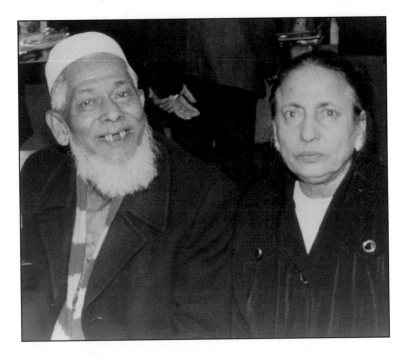

Plate 8: Bangladeshi couple, late 1990s

Source: Picture courtesy of the London Borough of Tower Hamlets.

1994–5 Survey of English Housing; a fifth of Bangladeshi flat-dwellers live above the third floor. It is also relevant to note (given the size of their households) that one in three Bangladeshis have no access to a private garden, yard or patio. Bangladeshis also stand out in respect of living in over-crowded accommodation. One measure of this is the so-called bedroom standard, which sets a standard for the number of bedrooms a household needs, depending on its composition and the relation of its members to each other. The standard is then compared with the actual number of bedrooms available to the household. Where the number of rooms is one or more below the bedroom standard, households are classified as overcrowded. Data for 1994 to 1995 indicate that nearly half of Bangladeshi households are below the bedroom standard compared with only 2 per cent of white households. Given this background, it is probably not surprising that the Survey of English Housing carried out in 1994–5 found 40 per cent of Bangladeshi people saying they were slightly or very dissatisfied with their accommodation. The figure for white households was just 7 per cent.

Migration history and background

Another important feature of the Bangladeshis is the nature of their migration history, which as noted is more recent than that of other minority groups, particularly in relation to completed families. The vast majority of Bangladeshis come from one particular district – Sylhet – and due to a process of chain migration, a substantial number appear to come from particular rural locations within this region. They speak various forms of dialect and the first generation at least had a low standard of literacy in standard Bengali. In respect of religion, the majority are Sunni Muslims.

A small number of Bangladeshis settled in Britain after the First World War, working as articled seamen from British ports. The largest group were to be found living in the East End. By the 1940s some had started the process of looking for employment in factories and restaurants in different parts of England. Choudhury records around 400 Bangladeshis from Sylhet living in London during the 1940s.[3] He notes that these early job seekers often found it difficult to find jobs in London, and that they began to find their way to the Midlands and also further North, working in heavy industry and textiles. In his book *The Roots and Tales of the Bangladeshi Settlers*, Choudhury gives the following description of life in the 1950s for these migrants:

In the earlier days, the ex-sylheti seaman settlers were middle-age, fathers or grandfathers themselves or they were in that age group. They usually did heavy industrial work. While at home they used to do shopping, washing, cooking and thus spent time in housework. The week days, if there was any time in hand, they sat with their praying mats and prayed or sat with friends and enjoyed talking while rolling paper cigarettes. They went to bed early to make up their lost sleep of the week days. At the weekend if they were not working, they used to visit friends or play cards. Those who had the habit of gambling went to the horse races or dog races. Many rather stayed at home and spent time in prayer and rest.[4]

Gardner notes of this period that it was a time of, as she puts it 'relent-lessly hard work', and she suggests this was a major factor in shaping the mens' identities.[5] In the 1950s, most still saw themselves as staying for a relatively short duration within Britain: they were 'sojourners' rather than 'settlers', to use Ballard's terms.[6] Gardner suggests that economic recession from the 1960s onwards had a major impact on the Bangladeshis, with many losing their jobs as labourers in manufac-turing and textiles industries. As a consequence many moved to London, seeking employment in the garment or restaurant trades. Even more significantly, an increasing number started to bring their wives and children to the UK. Gardner suggests that although changes in immigration laws were an important influence behind this last develop-ment, another factor was the extent to which the UK was seen as becoming a more acceptable place for Bangladeshi men to bring their wives and children:

> as the numbers of Muslims increased, and mosques, madrasas, and halal butchers were established they began to feel that their families would be more protected and catered for than previously. The 'snowball' effect was also important: the more Bengalis settled in specific pockets of the country, the more Bengali shops and services were set up, and the more comfortable people felt about their families coming to Britain.[7]

In this context, Inner London (and Tower Hamlets in particular) has become a major community for Bangladeshis. By 1996, they consti-tuted around 26 per cent of the population of Tower Hamlets. In all but two wards, the Bangladeshi group are the largest ethnic minority population. By 2001 they will form around half of the residents in

Bethnal Green. Clearly, in relation to thinking about change in the area, since the time of the baseline studies in particular, this has been a crucial development. What were some of the experiences and issues for the older people interviewed in our study? To explore this, we first summarise the characteristics of the respondents picked up in our survey of older people in Bethnal Green. We shall then examine their circumstances in more detail by way of qualitative interviews conducted with our respondents, along with other data gathered for this study.

Social characteristics of the Bangladeshi respondents

As noted above, elderly Bangladeshis comprise a very small proportion within this minority group. The 1991 Census identified 1,948 people of sixty-five and over, of whom eighty-nine were recorded as living in Bethnal Green. Survey data apart, relatively little is known about elderly Bangladeshis in the UK, although studies such as those by Gardner have begun to elicit some information. Data from studies such as the NSEM, and the Family Resources Survey, suggest high levels of deprivation in comparison with other minority groups, along with distinctive problems in relation to health.[8]

In our own survey there were sixteen men and seven women who had originated from Bangladesh. The majority (eighteen) were married, with four widowers and one single person. In line with the findings from survey data, the majority of those interviewed were members of large and complex households. Out of the twenty-three respondents, twenty-one had a child or children living at home. Fifteen of the households were of five persons or more (a similar figure, as we noted in Chapter 5, to that reported for all Bangladeshi households in the 1991 Census). Most of those interviewed were in rented (council-owned) accommodation. In nine cases housing was rented in the name of the respondent only; in two instances the respondent's son or daughter; in eight cases jointly between the respondent and their spouse; and in two cases jointly with a son or daughter. Income levels were generally low among this group with the majority receiving income support and housing benefit.

Respondents were asked a number of questions about their current health status and these confirmed studies such as those by Silveria and Ebrahim which suggested a range of physical and mental health problems among Bangladeshis.[9] Of the twenty-three interviewed, all but one rated their health as no better than fair, poor or very poor, and only one viewed it as good. Overall life satisfaction was low as measured by the Neugarten Life Satisfaction Index.[10] Again, this replicates findings from Silveria and Ebrahim who used an identical measure. They commented that the scores on this measure compared unfavourably with previous measures among the general population in other parts of Britain, including underprivileged London areas, using similar research instruments.

From this general description of the Bengalis, what information is there on their family and living circumstances in Bethnal Green? To discuss this we shall now consider the qualitative interviews with a sub-sample of those seen in the survey. The discussion will be divided into five main areas: migration histories of the sample; family structure; family support; housing and accommodation; daily life in retirement and old age; and feelings about Bangladesh.

Migration histories

The migration history of our sample is consistent with that recounted by Choudury, and by Gardner. In the case of men, most had come to the UK in the 1950s and early 1960s, although two had come in the 1940s, with the earliest in 1943. The majority had worked in a variety of places in England, typically in labouring work of different kinds. Mr Aziz is aged seventy and came to Britain in 1957. He starts to give information about his employment after talking about where he initially stayed in Britain:

Interviewer: Where did you first stay when you arrived in England?
Mr Aziz: I first stayed at Liverpool Street with my cousin's brother who lived there.
Interviewer: Then where did you live?
Mr Aziz: I stayed there for three years then moved to King's Cross. After that I moved to Luton to work in a plastics factory for one year.
Interviewer: What other jobs did you have?
Mr Aziz: I worked in a paper mill in Welwyn Garden City.
Interviewer: Can you remember any other jobs you had?
Mr Aziz: I can't remember the names of the companies.
Interviewer: Can you remember the type of jobs that you had?
Mr Aziz: Yes, I worked in a wood factory making sandpaper, and then a rubber factory. I also worked for the London Underground. My last job was in a garment's factory. [Mr Aziz goes on to describe a number of such factories in which he worked in East London.]

Later on in the interview, in response to a question about how Mr Aziz's life compares now with the sort of life he would have if he remained in Bangladesh, he comments:

> When I first came here I had to travel long distances by train to work and not just one train either; I had to catch two trains. I had to catch the 7.00 a.m. train, which meant getting up at 4 a.m. in the freezing cold. I did this by myself with some help from my cousin's brother. I had to learn the language slowly. Had I remained in Bangladesh, I would not have done this. I don't think many people in Bangladesh have done this sort of thing to earn a living, have they?

Mr Khan is aged seventy-eight and came to England in 1943. He describes coming to London by ship, staying for twelve years before returning for a period to Bangladesh, and then returning to work in different factories in London and the Midlands:

> I first worked in Hackney hospital. Then I worked for the Gas Board in Newham, then I went to Coventry and worked in an Army supply factory. There I had an accident and burnt my leg.

Mr Ali is aged sixty-nine and had been living in Bethnal Green for three years. He had come to Britain in 1967, and worked in a number of factories in the Midlands and the South of England:

Interviewer: Can you tell me where you first worked when you came here?

Mr Ali: I worked in Birmingham, then St. Albans, then Birmingham again, then in East London I worked in textile factories.

Interviewer: Did you have many friends in Birmingham, or people that you worked with?

Mr Ali: I had some friends here and there . . . but they all gradually left that area when they went back to Bangladesh to come here with their families.

Mr Ali's experience fits the pattern described by Gardner of men working for a period and then going back to bring their family to the UK, though now moving to London rather than the North or the Midlands where they had previously been employed:

Interviewer:	Can you tell me why you came to London?
Mr Ali:	When my family came to London, I decided to stay in London.
Mrs Ali:	When we came to London he (Mr Ali) thought it would be best that we remain in London. We were first put in a hotel for homeless families and we were there for five months. He (Mr Ali) has a sister in London so we thought it would be best to remain in London.

Mr Miah recalls a similar experience to that of Mr Ali. He is in his late seventies or early eighties and came to Britain in the 1950s. He describes his moves as follows:

Interviewer:	Where were you originally?
Mr Miah:	I was first in Birmingham. There I had many friends. I came to London because my eldest brother was here.
Interviewer:	When did you come to London from Birmingham?
Mr Miah:	About ten or twelve years ago. When I moved to London I stayed with my brothers and sisters, so we were very close. I was much healthier then and could travel. I was then placed in temporary accommodation in Wood Green before being housed in Tower Hamlets.
Interviewer:	How long were you in Birmingham?
Mr Miah:	I was twenty-one years in the same house.
Interviewer:	Did you have your own house in Birmingham?
Mr Miah:	Yes, I had a house attached to a grocer shop. But I sold the house and shop to return to Bangladesh.
Interviewer:	When was that?
Mr Miah:	In 1963.
Interviewer:	What work did you do in Birmingham?
Mr Miah:	Since arriving in England I've worked in factories, mainly as a manual labourer. I worked for the GEC company. That was my first work.
Interviewer:	Please tell us why you came to London from Birmingham?
Mr Miah:	I came for my family. When I came to London from Bangladesh with my family, my brother lived in London and wanted me to remain in London and not return to Birmingham. As he is my elder brother I stayed.

The importance of these migration histories concerns the issues raised by the discontinuities described by many elderly Bangladeshis. These are biographies marked by periods of separation and (re)unification with families, often adding to the problems encountered in old age. The complexity of people's lives is illustrated by Mr Ullah who had first come to Britain in 1948. His brother already had 'a little business' in Britain at that time. Mr Ullah worked with him for some time before moving on to work as an industrial labourer in different factories in the Midlands and in London. He recalls that during the Vietnam War he worked in a factory in London making various types of equipment for the war. He started this work in 1963 and he describes the 1960s as 'the golden years' when there was plenty of work available. When the company was taken over in the 1970s, Mr Ullah was made redundant. Soon after this, in 1978, he went back to Bangladesh, returning in 1980 to look again for work. His first son was born, in fact, about a month after he arrived back again in Britain. Mr Ullah eventually brought this son to Britain in 1982. He was joined later by his wife in 1986, but he returned often during the 1980s for short visits to Bangladesh ('coming and going to Bangladesh' as he puts it). He did eventually manage to get work again, being employed at a hotel in London from 1982 until compulsory retirement at sixty-five in 1995.

The history of this cohort of Bangladeshis is, then, one of complex attachments to different places within Britain, and to their own villages within Bangladesh. The industrial towns of Britain – Coventry, Birmingham, Leeds, Luton and elsewhere – were places where they went for work for money to send to their own families in Bangladesh. Rarely speaking English (virtually no Bangladeshis over fifty speak English as their main language) they were an isolated community, often lodging (as Choudhury study confirms) with other Bengali migrants. By the 1980s and 1990s, these early migrants were themselves reaching pensionable age, but in circumstances which contrasted in significant respects with the white elderly people within their locality. The fragmented nature of their life course meant that, for some at least, family life was at a point more characteristic of men in their thirties and forties than a group in its seventies and eighties. Migration histories had thus influenced both family structures as well as the type of support available, both resulting in major changes for people as they reached old age.

Household and family structure

Bangladeshis are typically described as having 'complex households'. Indeed, in this study (see Chapter 4) we have already referred to the extent to which the 'family groups' of Bangladeshis in Bethnal Green echo some of the characteristics of the extended family as described by Willmott and Young and Townsend in the 1950s. But the term 'complex households' is itself imprecise. It clearly refers to size of household, and more especially to generational depth. But these aspects alone may not sufficiently convey the sense in which such households may differ from other household types or the issues raised for older people by living in such households. Here, qualitative data, especially in the context of a largely non-English-speaking group, is helpful in unravelling some of the details and answering some questions about the nature of these family and household groups. Given that the idea of being surrounded by kin of different generations is seen as desirable, does it pose disadvantages along with some advantages? Are there costs as well as benefits as regards support? To start to answer these questions let us describe some of the features of the thirteen households on which we collected detailed information about different aspects of family structure and relationships.

Mr Ahmed lives in a three-bedroomed ground floor flat that was purchased from the local authority some seven years previously. This is a three-generation household comprising Mr Ahmed and his wife, four sons, two daughters-in-law and three grandchildren. Mr Ahmed brought his family to Britain in the early 1980s. He describes his early experiences in securing accommodation and contact with other relatives as follows:

Interviewer: When you came back with your family did you live in the present flat?

Mr Ahmed: No, no I lived in four flats in four months. I moved around wherever I could find suitable accommodation. I took private flats at first but did not find it suitable, sometimes because of the landlords. Then I applied to the Council, it was the GLC then.

Interviewer: The flats you lived in previously, were they in or out of Tower Hamlets?

Mr Ahmed: Inside. I was at a flat on Hackney road and then other places. It is difficult to always bring guests to this house because of the restricted space.

Interviewer: Could you tell us of any other close relatives you have in England?

Mr Ahmed: I do not have any close relatives in England. The relatives I do have are distant relatives. I have a relative that lives

	nearby but that's about it. There are my daughter-in-laws' families that live nearby, in Tower Hamlets.
Interviewer:	Are there any other relatives, close or distant, that you have regular contact with?
Mr Ahmed:	No, not really. There are a couple of people from the same village as myself in Bangladesh that live close by, with whom I have occasional contact.

Mr Hoque, in contrast, has a large network of siblings and other relations living in the local area. He lives on the third floor of a council-owned block of flats. This again is a multi-generational household comprising Mr Hoque and his wife, Mrs Hoque's mother, four sons (the eldest of whom was nineteen) and two daughters (one of whom is married with her own child). Mr Hoque also has three other married daughters, all of whom have children, whom he sees frequently. In the interview, Mr Hoque explained that he had a large family in London. He has three sisters all living in East London. His brothers have now died but he is in regular contact with his nephews (one of whom is living in the same block of flats). He describes his contact with his nephews as follows:

Interviewer:	Thinking about your nephews and your sisters, with whom are you closest?
Mr Hoque:	I am closest to my nephews. My nephews' fathers have all died so they come to me for help and advice. My sisters are busy with their families but they still think about me and I for them. Whenever I need to see my nephews, at least one of them will come. If my nephews cannot come to see me, then one of their wives will get in a taxi and come round.

Most of Mr Hoque's close relatives are now in England (with the exception of one surviving brother). He does, however, have a son-in-law still in Bangladesh. One of his daughters was married in Bangladesh (some twelve months prior to the interview) and she is still waiting for her husband to join her. This highlights an issue which was important to a greater or lesser degree for most of those interviewed, namely, the sense in which they were divided between families split between two different continents. In some cases, this reflected the existence of siblings and other relatives still in Bangladesh. In other instances, however, it was sons and daughters, either from a first marriage or from the existing marriage, who had been unable or unwilling to join them. An example of the former is sixty-eight year old Mr Bakht, who has been in England for approximately forty years. He lives in a fairly new house on an estate managed by a housing association. He is married with two sons (one of whom is married), and two daughters (both of whom are still at school). There is also an older daughter, now married but living in East London. However, Mr Bakht also still had important family ties with Bangladesh. At the time of the interview, he was severely incapacitated with a stroke and parts of the interview were conducted with his wife:

Interviewer: I would like to ask you about Bangladesh. Do you keep in contact with anyone in Bangladesh?

Mr Bakht: Yes

Interviewer: With who?

Mrs Bakht: His eldest son is in Bangladesh. You see he has married twice. From the first marriage he married my cousin's sister and had two sons and two daughters. Then he married me after my cousin died and I came to England with my five children. His eldest son from his first marriage is here and has children.

Interviewer: Does he have contact with the eldest son from the first marriage?

Mrs Bakht: Oh yes, they came round the other day to see him.

Interviewer: Does he have thoughts of going to Bangladesh to see his other children and relatives?

Mrs Bakht:: Yes, he sometimes talks about going back, which I can understand. He has his natural blood brothers and sons there, cousins and aunts are all there.

The existence of children living in Bangladesh was also important for Mr Ismail, a sixty-nine year old married man. He lived on the third floor of a three-bedroomed council flat with his wife and four children (aged eleven, eight, five and three years of age). Mr Ismail is in very poor health, and has had a number of heart attacks, as well as suffering from diabetes. He has seven children from a previous marriage, three of whom are still in Bangladesh and four living in the UK (one in the Midlands and three in London). The eldest son in Bangladesh is now aged forty years. Mrs Ismail describes the contact she has with her stepsons as follows:

They telephone occasionally, and we also phone. They try to keep informed about their father's health. They want him to go back to Bangladesh so that they can care for him, but I won't send him in this condition.

As we shall note later on, Mr Ismail had strong emotional ties to Bangladesh and he was clearly distressed at certain points in the interview when the subject of going back to Bangladesh was raised. In the majority of cases, the older men who were interviewed had lived in Britain for at least thirty years. On the other hand, the women interviewed for the study had invariably come at a much later date (usually in the 1980s or early 1990s). An illustration of this is the case of Mrs Naser. She is a widow who lives in a three-bedroomed house with her daughter (also a widow). The daughter has two sons living with her, one daughter-in-law and two grandchildren. She also has a married daughter living elsewhere in London, and another daughter in Bangladesh. Mrs. Naser is herself extremely frail, and suffering from a severe psychiatric condition. Her daughter describes her arrival in the UK and contact with relatives as follows:

Interviewer: So you are the closest relative to your mother?
Daughter: Yes.
Interviewer: How about your father?
Daughter: He died when I was young.
Interviewer: Who else does your mother have in the UK?
Daughter: Just me. My eldest son brought my mother here from Bangladesh by providing a sponsorship.
Interviewer: When did she arrive in the UK?
Daughter: About five or six years ago.
Interviewer: Before coming to the UK, who lived with your mother in Bangladesh?
Daughter: My other daughter in Bangladesh.
Interviewer: Does your mother have any close relatives in the UK?
Daughter: My mother has one step-brother. He lives in Oldham. There are no other close relatives.
Interviewer: Do you have any close relatives in the UK?
Daughter: No.
Interviewer: So you are the only child of your mother?
Daughter: Yes.

Most of these older people live, then, in households very different from those of the white respondents. These are multi-generational rather than single-generation households, in some cases with our respondents themselves having dependents still at school. For this, as well as other reasons, the issue of family support raised complex issues for these Bengali men and women. In the majority of cases, they were surrounded by relations from younger generations. But it would be misleading to draw conclusions from this that family support was automatically available or provided without undue pressure. In fact, as we shall see, in respect of informal care, this was a group facing considerable difficulties.

Care and support in the household

Many of those interviewed were, as would be expected from an elderly Bengali group, experiencing poor health, notably with strokes, heart problems and diabetes. Mr Bakht, to whom we referred earlier, had had two strokes, and was confined to bed at the time of the interview. His wife, who had come to England seven years previously, was the main carer, but she also supported her two school-age daughters and a son who had recently started college. She says that she gets some help from her children but also from her married daughter and her son-in-law:

Interviewer: Could you tell us what are the main things that your son-in-law helps you with?

Mrs Bakht: He comes round and spends time with his father-in-law, or might help feed him a little, and lifting him out of bed, into bed, into the chair, just generally being here at times.

Interviewer: How do you feel about the help that you get from your sons and daughters?

Mrs Bakht: They do what they can.

Interviewer: How do you think your husband feels about his care?

Mrs Bakht: He started to choke on some food the other night, my son rushed to help him and settle him down. I can't do all these things all the time.

Interviewer: Do you feel that you could do with more help in caring for your husband?

Mrs Bakht: I have been saying recently that if I had someone just to spend time with him while I was doing other things, that would be really useful, whether it was for two or three hours, it does not matter. The eldest son has gone to work, my son and daughters are at school and college and they'll be back late at seven o'clock. What should I do in an emergency. He is not eating or toileting properly.

Mrs Bakht is here raising the issue of the pressures involved in being responsible for caring for younger as well as older generations. She gets some help (Mr Bakht goes one day a week to a day centre for Bengalis) but still feels under considerable pressure:

Interviewer: Could you tell me how Mr Bakht spends his day?

Mrs Bakht: He sits mainly in bed. . . . One minute he wants to sit up then lay down, then move to the other side, that is all. So I have to do all that.

Interviewer: Does he have any particular routine or pattern to his day?

Mrs Bakht: No, he will eat when he says. I keep asking him what he wants to do or eat. Before the last stroke he used to read the Koran, but now he can't.

Interviewer: How often does he go to [the day centre].

Mrs Bakht: They come and take him every Thursday. They wanted to take him three times a week but now they cannot.

Interviewer: Do you wash him?

Mrs Bakht: Yes, every Thursday before he goes to the Centre I wash him. Then I clean him every other day.

Interviewer: How often do you change his clothes?

Mrs Bakht: About four times a day. Sometimes he spoils his clothes so I have to change him more.

Mr Ismail was another of our respondents who had a young family, and who was also in a very poor state of health with a severe heart condition. We noted that Mr Ismail had been married before and has four children in Britain. Mrs Ismail says she gets help when needed from her eldest step-son and the husband of her eldest step-daughter. She talks about their role in response to the following question:

Interviewer: Do any of your step-children visit in person?

Mrs Ismail: Yes, at least one of them will come once a week. One step-son visited yesterday. As you can see I cannot get out of the flat because of Mr Ismail, and he cannot go out because of his health as there are no lifts in these flats. There are times when I have to leave the flat, for instance when my children have to get to school. So at times I have to depend on my step-sons to help with things.

Mrs Ismail describes some of the things she does for her husband as follows:

Mrs Ismail: I have to bath him, take him to his bed and get him out. Feed him.

Interviewer: Does anybody come in to help you do any of these tasks?

Mrs Ismail: No, but somebody did come to look at me receiving additional welfare benefit for caring for Mr Ismail.

Interviewer: But you do not have a professional person coming to your home to care for Mr Ismail?

Mrs Ismail: No.

Interviewer: Have you ever applied for such a service?

Mrs Ismail: Yes, I did once when I had an operation. I was confined to bed and I could not look after Mr Ismail. My daughter phoned the local health clinic to tell them that I was unwell and could not look after my husband, but they did not send anyone round to look into the matter. Then my step-daughter and step-son-in-law helped out until I was better.

Some of the difficulties for these Bengali households occurred because of the range of problems affecting different generations. An example here was Mrs Khan, who was interviewed along with her husband. They live in a three-bedroomed ground-floor flat. Both are in very poor health and Mr Khan is confined to a wheelchair. They live with their three sons and one daughter, a daughter-in-law and one grandchild. The two younger sons, in their late twenties, are twins, both with learning disabilities. There is a fourth son, also with a learning disability, still in Bangladesh, who has been refused entry into Britain. The eldest son, who is married, is currently unemployed. Mrs Khan becomes distressed in the interview when talking about her son in Bangladesh, who she says has no one to look after him. In this situation, given the ill-health of Mrs Khan, the daughter-in-law and the eldest son were the main carer for Mr Khan:

Interviewer: Do you have problems with bathing?

Mrs Khan: Yes. I need help with bathing, my wife cannot help me. My daughter-in-law has to help me.

A daughter-in-law was also a crucial source of help for Mrs Naser, the widow whose household circumstances were outlined earlier. Her daughter describes Mrs Naser's health in the following way:

She is unwell in the head (a reference to a psychiatric illness).

Before she used to constantly speak, almost too much. Now with medication she speaks very little. Because of her illness she used to talk too much. After taking her to the hospital the doctor gave her medication and she now speaks less. . . . My mother cannot see or hear. She cannot speak or go to the toilet herself. One time she spent six nights in a hospital and I had to stay with her all the time.

However, the daughter herself is unwell and is unable to provide support to her mother. She says that: 'My own health is very poor. I take a lot of medication. I am unable to do any caring functions. I take tablets at night and at times my head aches for the whole day'. In this situation, the daughter-in-law (Mrs Begum) has become the key person supporting Mrs Naser. She came into the interview during a discussion about the value of day-centre help, suggesting, in contrast with the views of her mother-in-law, that this would be a good idea. Mrs Begum is twenty-five years of age and has two children. She expresses her views about needing help during the following exchange:

Interviewer: We heard from [your mother-in-law] that you are the main carer for your mother-in-law, her mother, and your own two children. Is this a lot of work for you?

Mrs Begum: Yes it is, but I have to do it.

Interviewer: What help do you think might assist you?

Mrs Begum: A day centre for my mother-in-law and grandmother sounds a good idea.

Interviewer: What do you feel about living in this house?

Mrs Begum: It is okay but we need more space and bedrooms.

Interviewer: What if a separate house was offered?

Mrs Begum: It would not matter as I would still have to look after them.

Other respondents who were in better health raised concerns about who would look after them if they became ill. One example is Mr Bokht who is seventy and lives with his wife in a council flat. He has three children (two daughters and a son), all still in Bangladesh. They have on a number of occasions tried to bring their son to England. Their concerns for their future without any of their children close by were expressed at a number of points in the interview:

Interviewer: Is your son married?

Mr Bokht: We went back and arranged his marriage two years ago.

Mrs Bokht:	We have tried to bring our son over but we failed. But if one of my son's children could come over at least that would be something. We are old; who is going to look after us?
Interviewer:	Do you have much contact with your daughters?
Mr Bokht:	Not really, they are with their husbands and they have many children. The eldest daughter has seven children. They have no responsibility to care for us . . . they have to care for their husbands and children.
Interviewer:	How do you feel when you think about your son?
Mr Bokht:	How do you think we feel?
Mrs Bokht:	Do you think we have any peace, knowing that our son is in Bangladesh?

Later on in the interview, Mr and Mrs Bokht are asked about the future in terms of who will care for them:

Interviewer:	As you get older who will you turn to for care?
Mrs Bokht:	We are already old, we have no one else. Other than our children, who else could look after us? You ask yourselves who could look after us; we have no one here.
Interviewer:	If you were ill, who might you go to given that your son is not here?
Mrs Bokht:	Then we would be in great difficulty. How would we get by? No one would take us like your own child would.
Mr Bokht:	Yes, that's right, how would we get by?

A major factor complicating the provision of support concerned the living conditions of these elderly Bengali men and women. National data confirms, as already noted, the extent of overcrowding in such households. Our qualitative data provides descriptive detail of the problems and tensions this brings to people's lives. Mrs Khatun lives with her daughter, son-in-law and grandchild on the seventeenth floor of a twenty-storey block of flats. She is very frail and was unable to converse without assistance from her daughter. In response to a question about her health, she comments: 'I have aches and pains in my joints. I have poor sight and I am always feeling anxious. I do not feel at peace. Because the flat is so high up I cannot walk out of the flat.' The daughter later explained that her mother's GP said she should go out and take regular exercise but that because the flat was so high up this was difficult. Mrs. Khatun commented that the lifts were always breaking down and that this meant that she couldn't go out. For some of those interviewed, the absence of any lifts in their blocks produced considerable isolation. Mr Miah lives on the third floor of a block of flats with nine other members of his family. He describes the problems in the following way:

Mr Miah: My real problem is not so much money but the fact that we live on the third floor and that I find it very difficult to climb stairs. Climbing down the stairs is not so much a problem, but climbing up the stairs is very difficult for me. Even though I hold on to the bannisters I still have to pause for breath. As a result of the stairs I do not get out of the flat as much as I would like to.

Interviewer: So the stairs are the main thing preventing you from going out more?

Mr Miah: Yes, sometimes I would really like to go out but when I think of the stairs I don't go.

Interviewer: Have you explained your difficulty with climbing stairs to the Housing Office?

Mr Miah: Oh yes, about fifteen times. I have visited their offices and written letters, but they have told me that I am low priority on the housing waiting list as they have many homeless people on the list. I have also explained that there are three people living in this house that are very frail. Myself, my mother-in-law and my wife. My mother-in-law has had an operation for the removal of stones as well as an operation on her eyes.

The absence of a lift was also a problem for Mr Khatun, who lives in a third-floor flat with his wife, son, daughter and two grandchildren. He has a major heart condition which restricts his movements:

Mr Khatun: I spend much of my time at home. I can't go out much as I sometimes get dizzy spells if I walk too much.

Interviewer: Do you get out to the local mosque?

Mr Khatun: No. Once I went and I felt very dizzy and fell over. I was later brought home by local people who knew me. I would like to go out but cannot.

Daughter-in-law: There is no lift in this block so my father-in-law has to walk up and down the stairs and that makes him dizzy. He could easily fall and hurt himself. We have explained that to the Council and they have put us on the waiting list.

Mrs Ismail commented in relation to her husband's situation (see pages 201–2) that: 'If we had a lift in these flats then it would be easier for him. At least he could just go downstairs and see the children off to school but he can't as there's no lift.'

For others interviewed, the sheer pressure of space was the abiding concern. Mr Hamid lives with his wife and seven children aged between seven and twenty-two years. They have five bedrooms. They are 'very small', Mr Hamid observes, and 'there is no storage space for any of our possessions'. Mr Miah also expressed concern about the pressures of space. Asked how many bedrooms in the flat he responds:

There are three bedrooms. My two sons with their wives stay in two rooms. I and my wife in one bedroom and my two youngest sons sleep in this room which is actually the living room. When guests come round we have to seat them here.

Later on in the interview he comments that: 'What would really help us out would be if my son was given a flat of his own nearby. He has one child. Either that or we were all housed in a bigger flat.'

Daily life and the role of religion

So far we have reviewed and described issues relating to the family structure and support of Bengali men and women in Bethnal Green. However, an important aspect of their lives concerned the role of religion, and especially the mosque as a point of reference and guidance in their lives. Many expressed frustration at barriers which prevented their participation in religion and prayer. These activities were especially important to these elderly men given that retirement seemed to bring very few benefits to their lives. Mr R. Ali said how he had found retirement hard to adjust to (in common, as we shall note in Chapter 10, with many of those in Bethnal Green), especially in the early days. He commented: 'In the morning what to do? No work, only get up, wake up, tea and what to do? Read a newspaper that is all.'

Accommodation problems were also important in restricting the movement of those in poor health. This point was made in the following way by Mrs Khatun in the following exchange:

Interviewer: When do your relatives usually visit?
Mrs Khatun: Usually to see me if I am feeling bad.
Interviewer: Which other relatives do you have in the UK?
Mrs Khatun: There are some relatives but I don't know where as everyone is busy with their lives.
Interviewer: Are there any people living nearby you here that you knew in Bangladesh?
Mrs Khatun: There are some that live in London, yes.
Interviewer: Do you have contact with them?
Mrs Khatun: Some contact, you always keep some contact that you knew in the past don't you.
Interviewer: How do you pass the time?
Mrs Khatun: I can't go anywhere because there are too many stairs to climb in this flat. What else can I do all day. I don't have much to do.

For most of those interviewed, family members and other contacts within the neighbourhood were central to providing structure and purpose to daily living. Asked to describe how he passed the time, Mr Miah highlights both these elements: 'I have a grandson from my daughter that lives here [and] I spend much of my time with him. There is also a local shop where I go every now and then to chat with the shopkeeper.' On the other hand, he comments elsewhere that he sees his relationship with his family as following distinctive boundaries:

Interviewer: Are there any occasions when your whole family get together?
Mr Miah: Yes, occasionally, on Eid and when my daughters celebrate their children's birthdays, but I don't get involved. Everybody respects me and my wishes in the family. I have thirty-three adult members in my family.

Mrs Khatun and her daughter talk about the importance of family gatherings in the following way:

Daughter: At times on special occasions we get together. On Eid relatives and family pop by.
Mrs Khatun: It is our culture that people visit each other on Eid and pay their respects or even inquire how I am, you understand that don't you?

Of great importance, however, for these elderly men was access to their local mosque. This is illustrated by the following responses by three men asked to describe how they passed their time:

> Well there is the mosque. I go there regularly. I don't go anywhere else. When you go to the mosque there will be some who you know and they will talk to you automatically (Mr Hamed).

> The mosque is the only real place I go for comfort and I meet people of my age whom I can talk (Mr Miah).

> I spend most of the time at the mosque. I go there five or six times daily. I work there on a voluntary basis and have done for the past eleven years (Mr Aziz).

Many of these men spoke with some pride about their own involvement with their local mosque and its development over the years. Mr Ullah, for example, commented that he goes every Friday to his mosque (the same one for the last eighteen years). He said that: 'He has a good communication going there'. Mr Ali commented that he had seen the present mosque grow from a small centre, and that he and others gave a donation every week towards improvements for the mosque. Mr F. Miah described his contact with his mosque as follows:

Mr Miah: We have a local mosque that will be opening soon in Bethnal Green. I am involved in its development.

Interviewer: Do you go the mosque now?

Mr Miah: It has not fully opened yet. We cannot pray there yet but the local shop nearby to the mosque has a basement in which we can pray. That is where I go for my Friday prayers. There are other big mosques in the area, such as in Brick Lane, but to get there I have to catch a bus then a fair walk. Because of my poor health I cannot manage the travelling. The new mosque will be ready in four or five weeks.

For those men affected by health problems, and restrictions through living in multi-storey accommodation, the difficulty of getting access to their local mosque was a real deprivation. The religious as well as social functions of the mosque were a vital element in their lives. For many, access was a major priority, ranking alongside the importance of family and relatives. Mr Ahmed expresses this as follows:

Interviewer: Do you visit the relatives that you mentioned, such as your daughter-in-law's family?

Mr Ahmed: Yes we visit on occasion. But there is little time to visit all the relatives as I spend most of my time at the mosque.

Interviewer: Do you like going to the mosque?

Mr Ahmed: Oh yes, I feel a lot of relief there and not only when I am praying.

Interviewer: So mentally you feel visiting the mosque does you good, how about your physical health?

Mr Ahmed: It helps my health also. It is a lot better than visiting other people's homes where all you will hear is talk and learn nothing, whereas at the mosque you can pray and feel good and it helps you rest.

Contact with Bangladesh and views of the future

A final area explored with our respondents concerned their feelings about Bangladesh and their thoughts about their future life. Our interest here was with how a group who were originally 'sojourners' viewed the prospect of spending their old age in Bethnal Green. How did their feelings compare with the type of situation described by our white respondents, as discussed in Chapter 5? Feelings about Bangladesh were inevitably complex and multi-layered for this group of elderly men and women. Bangladesh, and more especially their own particular village, was still a fundamental part of their memories and emotions. In some cases, this was given particular emphasis for men and women who still had close relatives, in some cases children, in Bangladesh. For almost all, however, life in Bangladesh represented a powerful and anchoring force, when compared with the perceived limitations of their current existence. But memories were often contradictory: people had strong feelings about their place of birth on the one side; but also remembered poverty, the lack of health care, and the sense of a disordered society. Mrs Khatun, who had been in Britain with her daughter for around seven years, expresses clearly this sense of uncertainty:

Interviewer: How do you feel now, having spent all your life in Bangladesh and now living the rest of your years in Britain?

Mrs Khatun: Maybe I will go back. But the doctors are not trustworthy. There is too much poverty. My health is too weak.

Interviewer: If you were in Bangladesh, do you feel you would feel better off?

Mrs Khatun: What can I say? Perhaps I would have been the same. There is no peace of mind anywhere. Bangladesh is poor. Doctors are very unsatisfactory.

Interviewer: Do you feel emotionally that you want to return?

Mrs Khatun: Partly, I will have no peace of mind wherever I will go, what can I say?

Interviewer: What do you feel about the future?

Mrs Khatun: It is up to God what happens in the future. I do think about the future whether I remain or pass away. The rest is up to God.

For Mr Miah, increasingly restricted to his third-floor flat, there were constant thoughts about returning to Bangladesh:

> One can never stop thinking about one's country of birth. Every now and then I feel for Bangladesh, especially as its so cold here and that I am confined to the flat. Also I would have had many visitors and many places to visit. You can never forget your place of birth.

Later, the interview returns to Mr Miah's feelings about growing old outside Bangladesh:

> Well, I can't forget Bangladesh although at times I am very critical of Bangladesh. [Mr Miah recites some phrases about having passionate feelings about one's place of birth.] Remember . . . I am living in a council house that does not belong to me. If I were living in Bangladesh I would be living on my own land. Isn't that true?'

For Mr Ali, with three children still in Bangladesh, there are more directly emotional reasons for returning to his place of birth. Now seriously ill, he is distressed at the thought of not seeing his children again. His wife comments: 'He really wants to go back to Bangladesh. When he hears of anyone going to Bangladesh he breaks out crying.' But most of those interviewed were also realistic about the differences between their lives now and what they would be like if they returned to Bangladesh. Mr Ahmed, now very ill, talked constantly of returning to Bangladesh, but his wife was clear that things were much better for them where they were:

Interviewer: What do you think Mrs Ahmed, do you think you would have been better off in Bangladesh?

Mrs Ahmed: No, there is so much poverty in Bangladesh. You are always hearing from people how bad things are.

Interviewer: If Mr Ahmed was in Bangladesh and was in poor health, how do you think you would have coped?

Mrs Ahmed: Well, we would not get the financial support we are getting now nor the medical treatment. Medicine in Bangladesh costs money and you cannot always get it.

Interviewer: Would you have more family support in Bangladesh?

Mrs Ahmed: Not really, because not all of them would have helped, plus I am getting help here that I would not have had in Bangladesh like the helper from the [day] centre, from social services [and] from the hospital, they provide all the help.

Mr Miah, who now has virtually no close family ties left in Bangladesh, provided a clear assessment of the advantages and disadvantages of going back:

Interviewer: Could you tell me how you feel about having spent so many years in another country? How do you feel about this country?

Mr Miah: It is good. I have few complaints about living here. You can live your life without much trouble, unlike Bangladesh where there are always problems. As long as you can work and get money then things can be all right.

Interviewer: How about from a health point of view?

Mr Miah: I think Bangladesh is better because of the warm weather, clean air and fresh food. Although we are eating plenty here you do not know what food is fresh and what is not. . . . Whereas in Bangladesh everything is fresh . . . we all have our own farms and the food is produced naturally. . . . But I cannot complain, at least we are living peacefully here and receiving health treatment when we need it.

Interviewer: If you compare yourself with a similar person in Bangladesh who do you think is better off?

Mr Miah: That person is more likely to be in poverty. If you look at my life, I was able to come here to find work to earn money to bring up my family and to buy things that I need. It is not easy to do this in Bangladesh because of the poverty. Then are those who are in business and have a good livelihood. Few people have the chance to be successful in business, but those who are live comfortably.

Mr Miah recognises that his own somewhat divided feelings about Bangladesh are very different from those of his children. He comments at one stage in the interview that: 'None of my children have been back to Bangladesh and they have no interest in going'. He develops this theme in response to a specific question later in the interview:

Interviewer: Do you expect your children to go back and visit Bangladesh?

Mr Miah: Not really. I brought them here when they were all young and all they have known is London. They would not know where to go in Bangladesh. Unless I take them back and fix up the house, otherwise where will they go and stay?

Interviewer: Do you regret that your children cannot recognise where you came from?

Mr Miah: Oh yes, very much. I cannot blame them for it but, yes, I would like very much for them to return to visit their home. If I get buried in Bangladesh, who will visit my grave?

These older people have now become settlers, most having worked for twenty or thirty years as industrial labourers in different parts of Britain. Families were eventually brought over; in some cases new families were started in early or even late middle age. Now in old age, these people are surrounded by often young families, but their own health is deteriorating. For them, memories were increasingly directed to their past in another country: 'their own place, their own birth place' as Mr Ullah put it. Bethnal Green is also still for them another country, one which they see as offering a better future for their children, even if it has brought rather limited opportunities and rewards into their own lives.

Bengali carers

Our study has confirmed the important role of Bengali women as carers for different generations within the family. For many of the women in the households described above, caring was stretched across the generations: support for an elderly husband (often twenty or more years her senior); care for children still at school or college; and care in some case for grandchildren. Evidence for pressure on carers is provided by data from the Tower Hamlets Bengali Carers Development Worker Project, which developed a profile of 235 such carers. Three-quarters of this group were women, with nearly half in the thirty-one to fifty age group. The majority were caring for people in the fifty-plus age group. Around half reported illnesses as a result of the pressure of caring, with stress and depression being especially common. In terms of the illnesses of those being cared for, in line with national surveys, stroke, diabetes, and heart problems were particularly common. To gain insight into some of the issues here, a focus group discussion was held with nine Bengali carers (all women), part of a carers group based at a day centre for Bengalis. Some of the difficulties faced by such women were brought out in a number of ways in the group discussion. Some of the issues concerned the physical tasks associated with caring for someone with a disability:

Facilitator: Could you tell me what problems you have in providing care?

Carer 1:   Of course we have problems. Lifting and carrying all day. Of course it is difficult.

Carer 2:   We get problems with our back, shoulders and other parts.

Carers 3 and 4:   We have to lift, push the wheelchair, feed and give medicine, we have to do the lot.

Facilitator: You told me you do everything by yourselves. Would any help from social services help you in your caring role?

Carer 2:   I do get help from social services but it is only for an hour. Sometimes in that one hour he does not need anything, no toileting or anything. So the helper comes and goes. One hour goes by very quickly.

But perhaps the most revealing aspect of these women's experiences concerned their vulnerability to threats of abuse and violence by their husbands. This emerged in a number of comments from the women. One carer described her husband's condition following a number of strokes: 'After his second stroke he could do nothing for himself. I had to do everything. Tower Hamlets Council did help me with some services.' In her description of the help she has received, however, she begins to raise other concerns:

What happened was that the hospital informed my GP and he spoke to the housing office who sent someone round to measure everything up. When they first fixed the rails my husband did not have the strength to use the rails. I had to lift him to do all the things he wanted to do but now, thanks to God he can use the rails. At the time my three sons were living with me. But at the time of my husband's first stroke my eldest son moved out. My husband would get very angry and would hit me or push me. Sometimes it would hurt me. Eventually my eldest son got married so that his wife could help me care for my husband. At the moment only my second son lives with me. My youngest son lives elsewhere. Sometimes when it becomes very unbearable I phone [the community centre] to send someone round to help me which they do. I think the fact he cannot do anything for himself and that he is sitting all day has affected him mentally, and therefore he becomes angry more frequently. Now things have not got better but worse. I have a lot of difficulty. His temper has got worse and he becomes angry more frequently. I cannot go anywhere out of the house. Sometimes he will just watch the television by himself, but if I watch the television he will hit me or get angry.

Later in the discussion, a women who had not previously spoken is encouraged to speak by the other women about her experiences:

Carer 6:   What can I tell you? He does not do anything for himself, he won't eat, sleep or change his clothes, he will just sit there in the same clothes. He will just bother me. Sometimes at twelve o'clock at night he will want to go out.

Carer 2:   You do not have any children with you?

Carer 6:   He won't sleep. He won't let me sleep and he will just bother me. Even when I'm tired and want to sleep he will bother me, and it is getting too much for me. He will eat at eight o'clock and then want to eat at ten o'clock, sometimes even interrupt me eating, so I cannot finish my dinner. I have to hide and eat.

Further on in the discussion the anxieties of the group come out in the following way:

Facilitator: This is something that is beginning to come out that you all feel very tense or frightened, that you do not know what will happen next.

Carer 2:   Yes, they have a worse temper now than before, it is as if they could kill you sometimes.

Carer 4:   Yes, they are still quite strong and he has a walking stick and threatens to hit you with it.

Towards the end of the group discussion, another carer describes her situation as follows:

> I don't know what he will do next. I never sleep comfortably, sometimes I feel he might kill me. I want to know how I can make him less bad-tempered with me. If anything ever happens to me he will have no-one to care for him other than social services.

There is a sense of great vulnerability among these female carers (most of whom are non-English speaking). Many convey a sense of isolation, despite their being members of large extended families in many instances. For these women, the extended family does exist and does provide some support, but much of the work and the pressure is seen to fall upon them as wives, daughters or parents. One woman spoke out towards the end of the discussion in a refrain which would find many echoes in different ethnic groups, and in many different types of societies:

> I want to say that within a whole family whenever someone falls ill it is up to us to care for that person, but when we fall ill there will be no-one to care for us. But also he is only bad-tempered with me not to any other member of his family. Why is this so?

In the conclusion to this chapter we pick up some of the issues raised by these women, for the next section of this chapter, however, we move on to discuss the position of Punjabi Indians in Wolverhampton.

Indians: the national picture

The Asian elders selected from the Wolverhampton sample were people who had migrated from the state of Punjab, which was divided between India and Pakistan in 1947. People from this area speak Indian forms of Punjabi and are almost entirely of the Sikh religion, although there are minorities of Hindus and Christians in the state. This section examines: first, the general demographic characteristics of the group; second, the migration history of people from India; third, the cultural and religious mores governing family life; and, fourth, some characteristics of the group interviewed for our research. The findings are also supplemented by a group discussion held with Asian interpreters and social workers employed by Wolverhampton Social Services.

General demographic characteristics

Overall, the Indian ethnic group displays a youthful population pyramid which does not begin to narrow until around the late-forties (1991 Census). Within this young population there is a marked excess of males over females, although (unlike the Bangladeshi population) women predominate in relation to older age groups. Indian people display the most elderly age structure of all South Asian ethnic groups. Nearly all those over the age of thirty-five were born outside the UK. In 1991, the UK-born were predominantly school age or young adults. Around two-thirds of both men and women are married, with divorce tending to be more common for Indian than Bangladeshi women. The English Housing Condition Survey (DoE) indicates 40 per cent of Indians living in council estates and low income areas. There is, however, a much higher incidence of owner-occupation than among Bangladeshi households.

The Punjabi family is of patrilineal descent and patrilocal residence, providing strong family-based support networks. Sons, for example, are responsible for the support of their parents; daughters-in-law are expected to provide practical support to their in-laws. Ahmed and Atkin suggest that younger generations of Punjabis may be providing extra services to their older relatives in terms of their knowledge of English culture.[12] In general, South Asian groups are likely to speak English, except among older people, where Gujerati is often spoken. In the 1992 Black and Ethnic Minority Health and Lifestyle Survey, only 20 per cent of Indian men and 10 per cent of Indian women aged between fifty and seventy-five reported English as their main language.[13]

Migration history

The main period of migration of Asians into Britain from India was in the late 1960s and 1970s. The 1991 Census recorded 840,255 Indians representing 1.5 per cent of the British population. A key destination for people from South Asia was the West Midlands, with Birmingham, Leicester and Wolverhampton, becoming important areas of settlement. In Wolverhampton, first and later generation Indians are spread across the city, but with particular concentrations in the inner city and adjoining districts. The attraction of Wolverhampton as an industrial centre, with opportunities for employment, was the motivating factor for men to leave India and set up home, later to be followed by their families. Mr Shaila, for example, came to Wolverhampton in 1963, and was joined by his wife in 1967. Four of his sons were born in India, the other four in the UK. There were exceptions to this pattern. One woman had emigrated from India as a 'dependant' when she joined another son in Wolverhampton leaving her husband and eldest son behind; another woman came with her husband to follow her Buddhist priest.

Mr Syal emigrated in 1963, exchanging a life as a high-ranking Government official with influence in his local community, for life as a labourer, renting on a council estate before moving into his own house. His wife joined him in 1969.

> I came in 1963, then six years later my wife came, our children were born in India and the youngest was six months when he came. I was employed at first making boxes and used to work seventy-five hours a week for £13 only. I came under a scheme where they paid you £5,000 and gave us a house to live in. . . . I was *surpanch* [village councillor] for the village, everybody respected me and I always helped poor untouchable people there. . . . My father too was *surpanch* leader for the village and a magistrate before that. He too helped others and had respect. . . . In India everyone knows me.

Despite his standing in India, he views his move as beneficial:

> There is no country like this one, the money you get now – this is the best country to live in. I have been to Canada, America and Singapore – when I was in the military – but it is better here.

All but one of those interviewed came directly from the Punjab to Wolverhampton and have moved around different parts of the City. Mr Singh came to Wolverhampton in 1954 and moved to several council properties before settling into his own house fifteen years ago. Since then, he and his wife have moved within the area, selling their property to his brothers as they came from India to work in Wolverhampton. Mr Syal lived in an adjacent street on arriving from India, and now lives in a house his children bought for him. One exception to this pattern was Mr Sangha who stayed in London for seven years before moving to Wolverhampton because of high house prices in the capital. Soon after moving his wife and children joined him from India. 'Houses were cheap here and we lived in another area before moving here when that house was demolished.'

Strong connections with India were apparent among our respondents. All had brothers and sisters as well as, in two instances, children from previous marriages living in India, and there were visits back, particularly for events such as funerals and in preparation for marriage by younger members in the household. Wealthier respondents owned or rented land or houses and, in one instance, a shop. Trips back, however, were infrequent (mainly due to the cost), with many revisiting India only three or four times during the last twenty to thirty years. Among wealthy families, yearly visits were made by the whole family. Families in India had particular expectations that their relatives in Britain would bring gifts and provide aid if needed. Roots were also maintained through marriage within Punjabi communities. One respondent, Mr Syal, said his main friends were still in India, despite his leaving there thirty years ago.

> I would like to go back and see them but I am not allowed to spend more than twelve weeks in India because they do not pay me. It is difficult to travel from Delhi to the Punjab as it takes one night. Twelve weeks are not enough as the travel time is long.

Although there were common features in the arrival of our sample group, fortunes had varied over the succeeding years. Mrs Bhatnagar, for example, came to England with her husband, who found work in engineering and the clothes warehousing business. They have kept a house in Noor Mahal, where they started a rug factory prior to emigrating, and return there every year. They now have a large house in Wolverhampton and have also purchased homes for their children. Others have done less well, experiencing a number of problems since leaving India. Mr Mumtaz came to England after the death of his first wife, working as a labourer in a plastics factory. In 1973 his son was murdered in a city-centre fight. A few years later, his twenty-eight year old son died of cancer. He now suffers from dementia and is housebound. His living conditions reflect his poverty, with rooms sparsely furnished, wallpaper peeling from the walls, faded upholstery, and a stench of urine.

Although many spoke of India, few contemplated returning permanently as they were embedded in their local Indian community with extensive ties of family and kin in the same locality. Mrs Lal, for example, returned to India following the death of her husband but later returned to be with her daughter. There was a general feeling among many of those interviewed that if they were to return there would be no

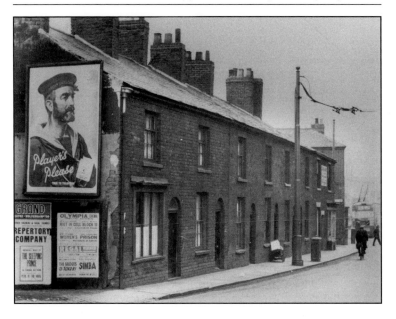

Plate 9: Heath Town, Wolverhampton, 1953

Note: This area of terraced housing was largely demolished by 1956

Source: © J. Dowdall, Wolverhampton Photographic Society.

one to support and care for them (a point also made by a number of Bengali men and women). Many people felt that their grandchildren in the third generation had little experience of India and did not wish to maintain links. Many girls, however, return in order to buy wedding attire (a source of family and generational conflict as families incur debt in the process). Many commented on the better standard of living in Britain (again echoing the comments of some of the Bengalis):

> This is the best country to live in. Life in the Punjab was better when I was there than now because of the fighting.

> It is difficult in the Punjab. They have to look after their own families. Circumstances in India are not good.

Mrs Bhatnagar, who returned to her home village annually, commented:

> We prefer it here. We do not like it in the Punjab. We do not get the

same facilities as here. We go and stay but we don't like it there and want to come back as soon as possible . . . If you become seriously ill, there is no one there.

Other respondents made similar comments:

We love everybody in India, but they do not feel the same way about us. They do not recognise if you give them something. They will cook for you. Then they will ask you when you are going back to the UK. . . . I never want to go back. . . . People treat you bad there. They are not very good. They say, 'whatever you have in your pocket hand over to us'.

We like it here. Better than India as we are on pension. Whatever we need we buy and eat it.

We get a lot of help from the Government and other facilities are available.

Family structure

Indians have among the largest households of ethnic groups in Britain. In the 1991 census 50 per cent of Indians were recorded as having dependent children, and 9 per cent living in households of two or more families; 21 per cent of the Indian population live in households with three or more adults and children, with just 3 per cent pensioner-only households. Our study confirmed this general picture; several households included great grandchildren as well as older people. In one instance, two houses had been knocked together so that two households could share in prayer and food together. An example of a multi-generational household was that of Mrs Kumar, who lived with her two daughters, two grandchildren, and her eldest son and daughter-in-law. Nearby lived her sons and their wives and children, numbering eighteen in total.

They work in the daytime, but in the night time they come and stay with me. They are always here to give me company. They cook and feed me since I have lost my husband and since my health is not so good.

Another respondent, Mrs Bhatnagar, reported: 'I live here with my husband and my daughter. My eldest son is here too. On the other side of the house is my daughter.' Mrs A. Lal had had ten children in all, five sons and five daughters. Of the five sons, one died at birth; two were twins and died at ages ten and eleven; her eldest son died approximately a year ago in India, and she has one remaining son who is planning to live in Canada. Of the daughters, two live in Wolverhampton, two in India, and one in Canada. Mrs Kaur lived with her son but had five other sons who lived in Wolverhampton. She commented: 'One is in Blakenhall, one in Oxley, one in Goldthorn Hill and the other two live locally. All my family are around me.' Others had more dispersed families in different parts of the Midlands. Mr Singh had two sons living in Leicester and Rugby and a daughter, with whom he had little communication, living locally:

> I have got two sons and one daughter. They are all married. Daughter has got five children, one boy and four daughters. The boys have got one of each child.We were all together before until they all got jobs, one in Leicester, other in Rugby.

Mrs Bhatnagar describes a similar pattern:

> I have got six daughters. One is handicapped who lives with me. One is in India but her two children are here. They work with my son in Manchester. I have two other daughters in Wolverhampton, one in Birmingham, and one in Manchester.

As the above example demonstrates, the extended family could be found locally but also with members dispersed across the country. There was also diversity in the mobility patterns of the second generation, with some moving to other predominantly Asian communities, in cities such as Birmingham, Leicester and Manchester, but others migrating abroad. Four families had sons or daughters living in America and Canada. Mrs Lal, for example, described her situation as follows:

> I have got five daughters; only two live in Wolverhampton, the rest live in India; one has gone to live in Canada and two of my grand-children have gone to live in Canada. Two nieces are in Canada. My nephew and his wife have gone to America as well as my niece.

The family was clearly regarded of great importance, and in one situation where divorce had occurred links were still kept between families. Mrs Kaur lived with her son following his divorce, but maintained links with her daughter-in-law and grandchildren; her other sons in India had married her daughter-in-law's sisters, and her closest friend in Britain was her ex-mother-in-law (who was also present at the interview). Mrs Mumtaz and her husband had previously lived with her son and daughter-in-law prior to their divorce. They moved to their current house to be close to both of them. Retaining links with family could also be a motivating factor in coming to England. Mr Amman commented:

> I have two boys and one daughter. My eldest one lives two houses after this. The youngest one lives further down the road and my daughter in the next street. They are all here as well as my grandchildren. I came in 1991, but my children came in 1967. My daughter came to be married and my son stayed, he was made permanent in 1973 and got married. She [the daughter-in-law] had a younger sister who got engaged to my younger son. We had no problem in India except none of our children were with us there. We wanted to stay but it was lonely without my children. The advantage of being here is that I can see all my children, we can see them going to school, laughing and crying. Our wish has been fulfilled.

Grandchildren were also important. Some households had grandchildren living in them, with our respondents taking on the function of main carer. Several of the older women in the study were looking after grandchildren while both parents were at work. Other grandchildren were older and were either in work or at University. Grandchildren were spoken of with much affection and were clearly of importance to our respondents even where they were living at a distance. Mr Syal said:

> All my grandchildren stay with me during the holidays. They like staying with me and I'm happy when they are here; they are our future. They all speak Punjabi. The younger one works in London. He is a computer engineer.

And Mrs Sangha commented: 'My grandson was born after sixteen years. This was very good news for me. My son was blessed after two daughters.' Regular visiting was mentioned frequently, and Blakemore and Boneham's finding that grandchildren acted as intermediaries between the Punjabi and English languages and cultures was also encountered in our study.[14] Grandchildren living locally visited almost daily, often helping out with shopping. In talking of grandchildren, older people were proud of the fact that they could speak Punjabi, although all felt that their grandchildren were unlikely to visit India, and had little desire to do so.

Caregiving and support

As with the Bangladeshi elders, poor health was a major concern which necessitated support from the family. The respondents without exception rated their health as poor, or very poor and many had mobility problems. Two of the men suffered from dementia. One woman was housebound because of knee problems and diabetes, another identified arthritis and asthma, others mentioned hearing and sight problems; these, complicated by language difficulties, rendered them housebound. Mrs Sangha had high blood pressure and needed the help of her daughter-in-law in the house; her husband suffered from asthma, blood pressure and diabetes. Mr Amman also suffered from high blood pressure and arthritis, while his wife experienced problems with her knees. Consequently they had moved their bed downstairs to avoid using the stairs. Mrs Kumar frequently suffered stomach pains, which hospitalised her on several occasions. Some of the women in the study were caring for husbands; one was paralysed (Mrs Kumar), another was insulin dependent, and another had heart problems (Mrs V. Kaur).

Despite the presence of large families to provide assistance, not all older people were receiving support. In some cases this was because there were few family members living locally, as in the case of Mrs D. Kaur, most of whose family had stayed in India. Mrs Lal had several children, living at long distances and a daughter close by but she considered her daughter too busy to help her: 'No she won't do it. She would have to leave the factory and then do my cleaning. She has fifty workers to take care of.'

Many of those interviewed retained their independence, making a major contribution to household tasks and the domestic economy. An example here was Mrs Kumari, who lived with her husband and eight others, looked after her unmarried sons, was the main carer to her four-grandchildren, and took in sewing to supplement the shared family income.

Caregiving tends, as studies such as those by Cameron show, to be a particular responsibility for women.[15] Among older women, the primary reason for coming to Britain was to care for their husbands.

Several, generally local studies, document the difficulties faced by Asian carers, including feelings of isolation and financial pressures. Blakemore and Boneham, however, argue that the Punjabis in Britain are in a state of considerable change, resulting in the marginalisation of older people within the family. Despite this, few older Punjabis lived alone, although there was evidence in the sample of older people not wishing to live with, and be dependent on, younger generations. Even where health problems precluded a reciprocal exchange of practical tasks, there was evidence of past support from older people in terms of caring for grandchildren. At the same time, patterns of caregiving within the household reflected traditional cultural and religious values, with women providing the main care, but with the decisions still in the hands of the male in the household.

Mr Singh suffered heart trouble, high blood pressure and diabetes and he considered it his wife's duty to care for him. 'My wife looks after me well and does not let me do anything. She will do all the washing.' Mrs Singh echoed this and described her day revolving around the needs of her husband and his mealtimes. Mrs Mumtaz described the some of the problems of being a carer in the following way:

> He does a lot of coughing and spitting where he feels like. I get fed up sometimes and swear. 'Why don't you and I die? You cannot control your mind and say things.' Just like a mother telling off her children. . . . He says, 'why don't you throw me out?' Wife says, 'where will you go.' 'I will go where people do not come back.' Then I cry and say, 'I am not going to throw you out.' . . . I am looking after him today. I don't know what's going to happen to me tomorrow.

Daughters-in-law were the main providers of care. The importance of bearing sons was highlighted in some statements such as: 'It is sad she has got all daughters. You know what it is like in India.' Daughters-in-law provided all practical household support, whereas sons were reported to visit to check up on their parents, take them out in the car, and do some shopping. There was a clear expectation that the family will continue to provide care. Mrs Kaur's daughters lived across the road (in separate households). At night (while their husbands were working on night-shift) they stayed with her for company; they also cooked for her. Mr Singh's daughters-in-law did all the work in the house, cooked and shopped for the food. They had also purchased his house. Where there were no daughters-in-law, daughters acted as substitutes, and where divorce had occurred, daughters-in-law still kept in touch. One man living alone (Mr Singh) was supported by his younger son, who washed his clothes and cleaned the house. His daughters had moved to Leicester and Yorkshire. Although grandchildren live locally they did not help out.

Daily life

Gender differences were also reflected in daily routines and living patterns. Women's activities were predominantly home and temple centred: listening to the radio, housework, gardening and visiting the temple. Mrs Bhatnagar, for example, has a bath after waking, does morning prayers, cleans, and plays cards with the family:

> I go to the city on a Saturday if my daughter-in-law insists, otherwise I do not go out. My daughter-in-law doesn't let me do anything. I go in the garden or have a walk and go to my daughters sometimes. My daughter (who is handicapped) goes to a day centre at 7.45 to return at 4.30 every day in the week.

Daily routines are often tied up with activities with her daughter or daughter-in-laws:

> My daughters come and visit. I get up at 5.00 a.m. or 5.30 a.m., have a bath, make tea, sit down and call for the girls to go to school. After she goes to school, I start tidying up. Afterwards my daughters come, they cook, clean and hoover the place. They come back and make lunch and we have it all together.

Mrs Kaur lived with her divorced son. In terms of activities, she visited the temple and spent time with her grandsons and friends. She did not go out at night: 'I just sit and relax. I don't do a lot.' Mrs. Kaur commented: 'I go and visit my children but I want to be home by 6 o'clock because I listen to *path* (evening prayers).' Mrs Sangha reported: 'I get up at 6.30 a.m. I make tea for my son, he goes to work and I spend the rest of the day tidying up or relaxing.'

Men were more involved in visiting the temple and in public activities. Mr Amman would wake at 5 a.m. to say prayers, then visit the public library each morning to read Indian newspapers following his visit to the temple. After lunch he attended the Community Centre, and then when the children returned from school he played with them. His wife spent most of her time in the house or with her sister-in-law.

Daily life, as some of these comments imply, also centred around prayer. Some of the women respondents were *Radhasaomi*, an ultra religious sect with strict dietary conventions. In all households there were portraits of gurus on the walls which were referred to as important sources of spiritual support. Mr Singh's daily routine followed strict patterns prescribed by his guru, including prayers at 3.00 a.m. for three and a half hours, and a visit to the temple after breakfast where he sits for two and a half hours. After prayer (*path*) 'I have my tea, I eat and lie down. My wife brings food. I am in bed by nine o'clock.' Apart from temple visiting, Mr Amman's other main activity during the week was visiting the city centre.

Apart from the local temple, few community facilities were visited and there was only limited contact with neighbours. Some respondents disliked the 'gossip' that took place in the community centres. Activities were family- and locality-specific. Friends were found in the temple. Even where people were described as housebound, the temple was mentioned as a place of importance. Where families had moved outside the predominantly Asian community they felt isolated from activity. Mrs Kaur commented: 'I liked it in Low Street. You could go to the shops and visit friends. It is very quiet here. I used to go to the shops and talk to everybody. Most of our people live in that area.'

Mr Mumtaz, suffering from dementia, attended a day centre to give his wife an occasional break. She, however, was housebound, and spent her day listening to the radio. She felt most of the things she did were boring and monotonous, and had a negative view of life in general, bordering on depression. Most respondents did not go out at night, because there was nothing to do outside at night or because they did not feel safe. Even during the day some feared walking to the city centre. Mrs Kumari insisted on her son phoning her every hour from work to check she was alright.

> I do not even know the shops. I might go with her (daughter-in-law), I do not even know the names of the road. I am scared to bring a bottle of milk from the Indian shop. I do not know regular money. I cannot go out on my own: I have hearing and sight problems. I cannot understand their language.

In general, though, the interviews demonstrated a clear expectation that the family would provide care in the future. This was borne out by one son, who was moving house to Leicester with his father in order for his sisters to take a share in the care. Residential care was not viewed as an option. In response to the question asked in all interviews, 'If you became seriously ill who would look after you?', all respondents opted for daughters or daughters-in-law rather than any form of residential care. Mrs. Bhatnagar commented: 'My daughter and family will support me. My daughter-in-law is very nice. My sons did everything and they will do everything in the future.' This was echoed by Mr Amman: 'The way I get support from my children, I am very happy. I'll wait and see what to do.'

Conclusion

The two groups discussed in this chapter demonstrated similar characteristics in the ways they translated their culture into a British context. Both Bangladeshis and Punjabis were surrounded by kin of different generations, either within the household or within close proximity. Cultural traditions and geographical proximity reinforced the caregiving roles of females within the family, and religion played an important role in daily life, particularly for the men in the study. Strong emotional links were retained with family remaining in India or Bangladesh, yet returning in old age to these countries was seen as unrealistic, particularly among younger generations. In other respects the two groups were distinctive from each other. The Bangladeshis are a younger population than the Indians. They are clustered in poor housing and are concentrated in particular geographical areas. In contrast, the Punjabis migrated at an earlier period, coming directly to Wolverhampton rather than moving around the country in pursuit of work. Their sons and daughters are now themselves moving to different cities in the UK, as well as abroad, in search of work and educational opportunities.

In comparison to our baseline studies, there is the continuity provided (as observed in Chapter 4) by vibrant kinship environments within which older people both give and receive support. But in some respects these environments also helped to conceal patterns of isolation and deprivation among ethnic minority elders, problems which seemed especially acute for those with poor physical and mental health. Here, perhaps the most striking continuity was with Selvon's *Lonely Londoners*, as highlighted in Chapter 2. This was especially the case with the first-generation Bangladeshis interviewed for our study. They would certainly echo Selvon's view that: 'Nobody in London does really accept you. They tolerate you, yes, but you can't go in their house and eat or sit down and talk. It ain't have no family life for us here.'[16] In fact, they had done their best to develop strong family ties but – as reported in Chapter 5 – 'toleration' had been slow in coming. They continued to experience the loneliness and sense of loss felt at some point by all migrants, but often felt most profoundly in old age when hopes of returning 'home' had finally receded. At the end of their lives, they sit in their house or flat dreaming of the children from whom they may be separated, and the village they will never see again. They are aware of the loss of one 'home' and perhaps a sense of rejection from the place where they have finally settled. This a very different old age from that experienced in our baseline studies, but one which seeks solutions in ways which would have been familiar to older people in those post-war years.

Chapter 10

The social world of older people

The experience of retirement and leisure

Introduction

So far this study has focused upon different aspects of social change as reflected in family and community-based relationships. However, another area of interest – and an important aspect of the original Bethnal Green and Woodford studies – involves what may be loosely termed the 'social world of older people'. One element here – powerfully described by Peter Townsend – was the crisis faced by elderly people (men especially) when faced with the loss of work. A central argument in his research was that for working-class men retirement was 'a tragic event', one which had major repercussions for all aspects of an individual's life. Few among those experiencing retirement in the 1950s seemed able to occupy their time in ways that gave satisfaction:

> Reading, walking in the park, visiting their children, listening to the radio, tending a few flowers, occasionally going to a club or cinema or an outing to Scotland – these seemed to be common recreations of retired men. They did not give much opportunity for self-expression. Those unable to help their wives or female relatives in domestic and family activities were left without many means of justifying their lives. . . . This is why so many men talked of retirement as a tragedy. . . . Their life became a rather desperate search for pastimes or a gloomy contemplation of their own helplessness, which, at its worst, was little better than waiting to die.[1]

The situation of women, on the other hand, was viewed differently. Although more than half of those interviewed had been employed in the years preceding retirement, this was seen as less important in respect of their status and standing within the community. Women, in contrast with men, were seen to be embedded within a network of family relationships, which assisted social integration in old age. This was reinforced by the idea of the home as essentially female territory, where (as noted in previous chapters) the male was a marginal figure when faced with the close bond between mothers and daughters. Townsend describes this as follows:

> Some men were able to take on some of the domestic chores, particularly if their wives were infirm and had no daughter available, but many found even this unnecessary. Competent wives and competent daughters did not need them in the home. 'The wife always used to have the place on her own. They get grumpy if you get in their way. "I want to do this", she'll say. "What are you doing here?" and you have to get out . . . you see some of the old 'uns. It's like penal servitude. They come out about nine in the morning and don't go home till five in the afternoon.'[2]

Loss of income was important in placing restrictions on people's lives, depriving men in particular of the status of breadwinner. But the suggestion from Townsend's work was that the crisis of retirement was about more than money (or the lack of it). Work had given people a sense of feeling needed and wanted; retirement, in contrast, seemed to make many feel useless and ill at ease with themselves. This finding was also referred to in the original Woodford study where, among the working-class older men interviewed, similar experiences were reported in some cases. However, Willmott and Young emphasised that these were in fact the exception; working-class men, though certainly worse off than the middle class, were like them in a number of respects. In particular, there did not seem the same sense of exclusion from the home:

> On the contrary, the [men's] relationship with their wives is a close one. 'Partnership' has gone further in Woodford than in the East End, among the older married couples as among the younger. Woodford fathers and mothers more often own their homes and have gardens to tend, and the interest in the house and garden is something the couples hold in common. . . . The old people of Woodford, in all classes, seem altogether to have a more companionate conception of marriage. . . . This . . . is specially evident in retirement.[3]

The sense of partnership between husband and wife was reinforced by differences in kinship patterns between Bethnal Green and the suburb. In the former, daughters remained close by from their wedding day onwards, complicating the relationship between husband and wife. In the suburb, parents and children led separate lives: husband and wife developing common interests of their own, rather than activities focused around their children. These differences were reflected in leisure attachments. While Townsend had relatively little to say about leisure activities, implying that these were work rather than community-based, Willmott and Young stressed the importance of 'organised sociability' in the suburb, an active social life often being used to replace the gap created by the absence of relatives:

> The older men belonged to the bowls or golf club, the Conservative Club or the Rotary. Mr Coote told us, 'I go along to the bowls club nearly every day in the summer'. Mr Cutbertson said, 'I go to the golf club about three times a week. I belong to the Woodford Wells Cricket and Tennis Club as well. I used to play cricket and my wife played tennis – we don't play now, but we still support the club. We always go to the cocktail party at the beginning of the season, and usually to one or two of their other functions'. Mr Cooney belongs to the golf club, the bowls club, the Essex Beekeepers' Association and the Conservative Club: 'I'm not strongly political. I go over there to play snooker two or three times a week.'[4]

These were, as the researchers observed, somewhat selective organisations, often excluding (or appearing to exclude) working-class residents of Woodford. None the less, their importance raised implications for our own study in respect of whether this type of 'sociability' retained its significance in retirement. Moreover, there was also the issue of the extent to which the retirement experience had itself changed in these localities, since the baseline studies. Had family life and family support become less important, given more positive views about retirement as a valued stage in the life course? Had leisure and related activities began to supplant those built around the immediate and extended family? These are some of the questions to be explored in this chapter.

The transition to retirement

In the 1950s, for working-class men in particular, a strong work-based culture existed alongside that of family ties and relationships. This undoubtedly reflected the necessity of work given the low level of state benefits (a point graphically illustrated in Townsend's study). However, it also illustrated the absence of a concept of retirement within working-class culture, a point developed in Peter Stearns' research on old age in France, but one also applicable to Britain.[5] In the 1950s, a large proportion of men continued to work after the age of sixty-five. Of the sixty-four men interviewed by Townsend, nineteen were in full-time work, with a further six in part-time employment. Many more expressed a desire to find or return to work if at all possible. Among the women interviewed, four (all widows) were in full-time employment, and a further twenty worked part-time.

Fifty years on, our own sample of 627 older people reflected the institutionalisation of retirement over the post-war period. Out of this group, 85 per cent considered themselves wholly retired. Only a small proportion – 7 per cent of men and 5 per cent of women – had been in paid work in the week before the interview. In relation to the areas, while 61 per cent of Townsend's men had been wholly retired, the figure in our study was 87 per cent (the figures for Wolverhampton and Woodford were 80 per cent and 81 per cent). For women, while 17 per cent in the original Bethnal Green study were employed, the figure from our sample was 3 per cent (the figures for Wolverhampton and Woodford were 5 per cent and 2 per cent). On the other hand, virtually all of those interviewed had worked at some point over the life course: all the men and most of the women (90 per cent) had been in paid work at different times (among women this was the case with 97 per cent of those in Woodford; 87 per cent in Wolverhampton and 86 per cent in Bethnal Green). Among those who had worked and subsequently retired, the total sample divided evenly among the 48 per cent who had retired at or soon after pensionable age, and the 51 per cent who had finished work at some point before pensionable age. The mean age of retirement for each of the three areas was roughly similar, except for Bethnal Green where women had a later age of retirement – fifty-seven compared with fifty-two for women in Woodford and Wolverhampton.

The transition to retirement often shows marked variations in respect of the reasons given for leaving work. The study of retirement and retirement plans by Bone *et al.* found that the commonest reasons given for taking or expecting to take early retirement were to do with ill health, being offered a reasonable financial inducement, wanting to enjoy life while still young and fit, and wanting to spend more time with the family.[6] For men in this study, among those who had retired from work, 43 per cent cited their own ill-health as one of the factors behind the retirement decision. For women the figure was 31 per cent; 35 per cent cited a financial inducement (compared with 10 per cent of men). Our study used similar questions about retirement to those of Bone and her colleagues.

Informants were shown prompt cards from which they selected from a variety of reasons identified in the retirement literature for leaving work. For men going before state pension age, early retirement was a factor listed by one in four. One in three listed health factors, but this was more common with the Bethnal Green and Wolverhampton sample (40 per cent and 37 per cent respectively) than for those in Woodford.

Among women, out of the thirty-two going before state pension age, fifteen (47 per cent) list a health reason (the comparable figures for the other areas were ten (12 per cent) in Woodford and seventeen (25 per cent) in Wolverhampton). Among people who had left work at or after state pension age, two-thirds of the men cited a fixed retirement age. There were clear differences, however, between the areas, with 74 per cent citing this in Wolverhampton compared with 54 per cent in Woodford (the figure for Bethnal Green was 65 per cent). Finally, in the case of women, a fixed retirement age was again the most important reason, but was cited by only 38 per cent of respondents overall (Wolverhampton again stood out at 51 per cent). In Bethnal Green, 27 per cent of women cited ill-health as a factor in their retirement, compared with 19 per cent of women in Woodford and 13 per cent in Wolverhampton.

Experiences and perceptions of retirement

As already discussed, Townsend's study was of considerable influence in highlighting the importance of paid work for men, notably as a means of integration within the community. People spoke of losing part of their identity in moving away from relationships and attachments within the workplace. This was seen to provoke anxiety, even a sense of fear, among many of those interviewed. To what extent had this changed in the intervening years? What evidence did we find for the growth of more positive attitudes to retirement? One way of examining this is to consider the type of image which people have about a period such as retirement. Is it, for example, seen as a new phase in life? Alternatively, do people view retired life as rather similar to the one they had when working? We presented people with five phrases describing retirement and asked them to identify which best summarised their own views (Table 10.1). Overall, the most popular (with 44 per cent of respondents) was the notion of retirement as a 'new phase in life'. This was consistent across the areas both for men and women, except for Bethnal Green, where fewer people could identify with this view. Men (and to a lesser extent women) in Bethnal Green were much more likely to view retirement as the 'beginning of old age' (40 per cent did so). At a further

Table 10.1 Images of retirement

	Wolverhampton		Bethnal Green		Woodford		Total	
	n	%	*n*	%	*n*	%	n	%
An extended holiday	32	15	33	18	33	17	98	17
A new phase in your life	104	50	50	30	103	52	257	44
The beginning of old age	38	18	56	31	30	15	124	21
A life rather similar to the present	15	7	18	10	16	8	49	8
A rejection by society	7	3	11	6	0	0	18	3
Can't say	13	6	11	6	18	8	43	7
Total	209	100	179	100	200	100	589	100

extreme, a small group saw retirement as a 'rejection by society': none in Woodford but eleven (6 per cent) of those in Bethnal Green, and seven (3 per cent) in Wolverhampton.

What links can be drawn between the images identified in Table 10.1 and experiences of work and retirement? Let us examine, first, the issue of work and relationships at work. A substantial proportion of those who considered themselves retired were still in touch with people with whom they had previously worked (46 per cent). However, this was less true of the Bethnal Green sample (37 per cent) than the other two areas (50 per cent in each), despite the fact that individuals were more likely to have had their usual job in or around Bethnal Green itself. The extent to which people felt a sense of loss about workplace contacts was explored by asking individuals whether they missed being with other people at work. Evidence that this could be an important issue for retired people was noted in a survey by Parker conducted in the late 1970s, which found 36 per cent of retired men and women saying that losing the company of people at work was what they missed most about their job (a finding which applied rather more to women than it did to men).[7] Overall in our research, 41 per cent of those interviewed reported missing other people from work, with no differences between men and women on this issue.

There were no differences between the areas, with the exception of Bethnal Green where women (in comparison to women in the other two areas) were more likely to report that they missed these contacts: of the eighty-seven women who considered themselves fully retired, forty-five (52 per cent) indicated this compared with around one-third of the women in Woodford and Wolverhampton.

Another important question concerns the extent to which people feel they have difficulty keeping occupied in retirement, an issue which was of great concern to older people in Bethnal Green in the 1950s. Our findings on this issue come from a number of sources. First, we asked the direct question: 'Have you found times since your retirement when it has been difficult to keep occupied?' Overall, around a fifth (22 per cent) of those interviewed indicated that this had been the case, with a greater proportion of men reporting this than women. Men in Bethnal Green were much likely to report problems than those in the other two areas (42 per cent did so compared with one-fifth of men in Wolverhampton and Woodford). However, this was also the case with women in Bethnal Green, where around one-third of retired women (31 per cent) had difficulty keeping occupied compared with 19 per cent of women in Wolverhampton and just 8 per cent of those in Woodford.

We then asked the question: is there anything you particularly like or dislike about being retired? Interviewers could also record 'nothing about retirement that respondent dislikes'/'no pleasure in retirement' to use where appropriate. Examining aspects of retirement that people liked first of all, there were two main clusters among men. Around one-quarter (23 per cent) highlighted having the time to follow their own interests, while 17 per cent mentioned freedom and independence; 9 per cent spoke of having time to pursue hobbies. The issue of independence, however, showed some variation across the areas, with one-fifth of those in Wolverhampton and Woodford reporting this compared with 10 per cent of men in Bethnal Green. In line with this, while 27 per cent of men overall could identify nothing they especially liked about retirement, this was more characteristic of those in Bethnal Green (42 per cent in comparison to one-fifth of men in the other two areas). Among women the same clusters appeared but with the 'time to do your own thing' being more prominent (35 per cent overall) with the freedom of retirement being the next most popular (14 per cent). Again, there was an area difference here with only 6 per cent of women in Bethnal Green identifying with this, compared with 18 per cent of those in Woodford and 16 per cent in Wolverhampton. The same pattern appeared regarding 'no pleasure in retirement', with one-third (33 per cent) of women in Bethnal

Green indicating this, in comparison with 12 per cent of women in Woodford and 16 per cent in Wolverhampton.

Turning to 'dislikes about retirement' we first have to start with the point that overall 41 per cent of men reported that there was nothing they disliked about retirement. Again, there was an area difference here with 51 per cent of men in Woodford indicating this, compared with 36 per cent of men in the other two areas. The only issue which got beyond double figures was that of boredom (identified by 13 per cent) and this was clearly a bigger concern in Bethnal Green (reported by 20 per cent of men) than the other two areas. The pattern was roughly similar for women with 54 per cent disliking nothing, but again women in Woodford registered a higher figure (65 per cent) in comparison with Wolverhampton (54 per cent) and Bethnal Green (42 per cent). One-fifth of women in Bethnal Green identified financial problems as a major concern; 12 per cent mentioned boredom. In Wolverhampton, there was a small group of women (8 per cent) who identified problems of loneliness.

In many respects these findings do suggest important continuities with the earlier studies. In Bethnal Green, in the 1950s, time often seemed difficult to manage for retired people; forty years on, similar feelings seem to be voiced:

> I'm on my own now and my son helps out but I've got too much time on my hands (seventy-six year old widowed man).

> I've worked hard and I get bored. It can get a bit lonely at times (seventy-six year old married man).

> Just have too much time on my hands now. I am fit for my age, not enough to occupy me (seventy-three year old married woman).

> Not doing anything. Bored (seventy-two year old single man).

> Unable to do things I used to do. Feel kind of useless (sixty-six year old single woman).

Running through the comments were also concerns about money; of constantly living close to the margins, and being denied much in the way of choice. In the earlier survey, one of Townsend's respondents, Mr Kite, expressed this experience as follows:

> I used to go out and see the boys on Saturday evenings. I'd meet my

sons-in-law and we'd go out to the pub. . . . Now I can't do it. It's like being a pauper. I had to turn away from that because I didn't have a pound like I did in my pocket. I couldn't stand anybody anything (drinks). I couldn't do my share.

Some of our Bethnal Green respondents reported similar concerns:

Miss having money. I can't do what I want. I enjoy going down to the pub but I can't afford it, only at weekends (eighty-three year old married man).

Loss of money. Boring sometimes when you're on your own. Just go to bed, that's it (seventy year old widowed woman).

The whole thing. When you go to work you have a system . . . you have money . . . you can buy and replace . . . now you can't . . . food and flowers. You just can't buy what you want not even necessities (seventy-three year old married woman).

Money. Living dead to the line. Can't afford to go out. Not having a garden where you can relax. Living here is too noisy but you cannot really go too far apart from using bus passes (sixty-four year old old married woman).

Not having things that other people have, like a car and holidays. I wanted to go to Clacton but the train fair was £15 each so we couldn't go (seventy year old married man).

This last comment is a reminder of the difficulties of a working-class group where very few have access to a second pension or savings of any substance. This was equally true of some of the respondents in our other areas, but it was certainly given a much stronger focus in Bethnal Green. Correspondingly, where people did focus on the benefits of retirement, these often emphasised the reward of not having demands placed upon one's time. Wolverhampton and Woodford respondents were also similar in this regard and a selection from all three areas is brought together below:

You can do what you like. You can go out and meet people. You don't have to worry about getting about in the morning (seventy-seven year old widowed woman, Bethnal Green).

Being lazy. Doing what I want. Doing my own thing (seventy-three year old married woman, Bethnal Green).

You can do things in your own time. Before I had to get up in the morning, do the ironing, do the housework. Now you do it in your own time (sixty-four year old married woman, Bethnal Green).

I seem to have more time for pleasure if I want it. I don't have to think about getting up. My mind doesn't have to panic about what I will find when I get [to work] (sixty-five year old married man, Wolverhampton).

Your time is your own and you can get up and do as you please nothing planned (seventy-five year old single woman, Wolverhampton).

Being able to lie in bed in the morning . . . not having the pressure of getting up in the morning. Come and go and stay out for the day if I want to (sixty-eight year old single woman).

It's a permanent holiday. After the hassles of travel it's a pleasure not to have to go to work (eighty-three year old single woman, Woodford).

Yes, the fact that I don't have to get up in the morning and fight to get on the train and fight to get home in the evenings (seventy-one year old married woman, Woodford).

Get out when you want to. You can have time to watch Wimbledon (seventy-two year old married man, Woodford).

Underlying these comments there is one important change, at least from the type of reports in Townsend's study. For some of these retirees, there is clearly less guilt and worry about an excess of time or about not having the kind of responsibilities associated with work. That this was still an issue for a substantial group in Bethnal Green almost certainly reflects the poverty of the majority of pensioners in the area, as well as the impact of some of the changes to family and community life discussed in earlier chapters. The negative side to retirement was illustrated in other ways in our interviews. Especially striking here were a number of people in

Wolverhampton who spoke about the loneliness that seemed to run alongside being retired:

> Sometimes I am lonely. I missed the people I worked with (seventy-three year old married man).

> I am a little lonely since my wife died. Retirement means getting old and I don't want to get old (seventy-one year old widowed man).

> Yes, it gets a little lonely at times. It would have been better if I was married. I've always been a solitary bloke. Enjoyed my company over the years but still lonely (seventy-five year old single man).

> The loneliness. There's no real challenges and no motivation. I have to create my own challenges and motivation and I've got too much time (sixty three year old married woman).

> Get bored and lonely. Quite frightened being alone (seventy-three year old widowed woman).

> Loneliness. It's a lonely life (seventy-three year old widowed woman).

> You slow up when you get older . . . lonelier since my husband died especially (seventy-one year old widowed woman).

The comments from older people in Wolverhampton partly reflect problems of adjusting to living alone after a long period of marriage, again an important change here from the baseline studies. However, another side to this is people talking about the benefits of retirement precisely because it allows greater time for couples to spend more time with each other. The descriptions here are rather different from Townsend's in the 1950s but they do build upon the type of relationships described by Willmott and Young. They argued, as noted earlier in this chapter, that 'partnership' had gone further in Woodford than in the East End, and there was certainly some evidence for this from our own study:

> Yes. When we were both retired and, well, we did modern sequence dancing and we had lots of friends – they are all nearly dead now. It was the best time of our lives and visiting the grandchildren – we went touring in the car to Scotland and Wales (eighty-six year old widowed woman).

Both enjoy it – having husband home all day – we like the same things (sixty-two year old married woman).

Now that my husband's dead I've got to make up my mind and there's a void – but when he retired I don't think there was anything I didn't like about retirement (seventy-four year old widowed woman).

You can please yourself. Husband and I can spend more time together (sixty-four year old married woman).

Able to use my time as I want it. Able to spend time with husband and take up my hobbies (sixty-nine year old married woman).

Another development – again almost certainly a change since the baseline studies – is a greater self-consciousness, a sense of the disadvantages of ageing (rather than retirement), and the changes it brings in relationships with other people. Two respondents in Woodford complained about 'people talking to you like an imbecile' and 'taking you for a fool and thinking you are a bit soft in the head'. And people in this middle-class area talked rather more about how they 'disliked getting older'; physical change was happening at an accelerating pace, and for the first time (for this middle-class group) it was something quite unplanned and unprepared for. As one person expressed it: 'I'm getting old. I know that happens to all of us but nobody tells you what it will be like.' And there are darker fears which come through, triggered off by simple questions about what people dislike about retirement. The one line comment in a survey speaks volumes for the quiet desperation which still affects a minority of lives. An eighty-six year old woman (again in Woodford) sums up her present life with the terse comment: 'Lonely – just waiting to die'. And a seventy-five year old single man (also in Woodford) observes: 'Nobody that I know cares about me. I lost my family in the war and there's no one else.'

These are minority comments, and for each one there are many more which are reminders of the positive changes which retirement can bring. One aspect of the improvements since the baseline studies has been the growth of social and leisure activities in retirement. What do our findings tell us about changes since the baseline studies on this issue?

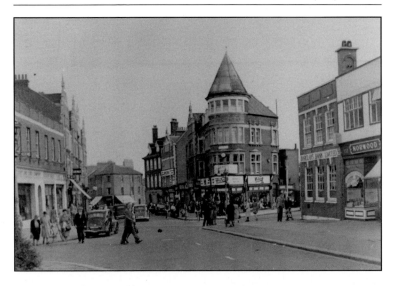

Plate 10: Shopping in South Woodford, early 1950s

Source: Picture courtesy of The Francis Frith Collection.

Leisure in retirement

A key change since the 1950s has been the transformation in retirement lifestyles. The baseline studies reflected a generation of older people who were largely unprepared for retirement, had not really expected to retire in many cases, and were certainly anxious about the change it had brought to their lives. The households of older people would have had few of the consumer goods now taken more or less for granted; very few pensioners would have had a television or a telephone, to take two examples. Leisure would have been shaped by the daily round of relationships within the family; alternatively, there were the ubiquitous social clubs for the old developed in many towns and cities (and in all three areas in our study) from the late 1940s onwards. This was an era of coach parties to the seaside, drinking in pubs and working-mens clubs (for men at least), visits to the cinema, football and cricket matches, and sitting in parks and greens. As Glass and Frenkel observed in Bethnal Green in the late 1940s:

> But if you walk into one of the few 'village greens', on a pleasant day, Victoria Park Square, Meath Gardens or St Matthew's Churchyard, you will soon realise that Bethnal Green is not all drabness and monotony. Between 10.00 a.m. and 11.00 a.m. about

> every seat is occupied by the old men. From then till lunch time they give way to the old ladies, who, in turn, are followed by the mothers and babies.[8]

Retirement was, then, shaped for men by their talking in the street and in pubs with other men; for women, it was the importance of home and street, in the company of other women (and children) within the family. How had this pattern changed in the intervening years? What evidence was there for a new world of leisure among our respondents? To find evidence for this we used a similar approach to that used in assessing the kind of relationships people felt were important in their daily lives. This time, however, respondents were invited to think about all the things that were significant in their life, whether they were 'social or domestic activities, hobbies or anything else'. They were asked to indicate up to ten different activities on a similar circle diagram to that used to identify social networks. Additional questions were asked about the first five named activities: where they were done? How long they had been pursued for? Who, if anyone, were they done with? Let us now consider what the information our respondents provided tells us about the social world of older people at the end of the twentieth century?

Most respondents (96 per cent) were able to show a variety of activities that they regarded as important to them in retirement. Between them, these respondents listed a total of 139 different activities, ranging from conventional social, sporting, hobby, educational and religious activities, to the home computer buff, the stained-glass window maker, the radio ham, the political activist and the 'people watcher'. Our respondents confirm that leisure, as defined by older people, can encompass a vast range of activity. Leisure in this sense, is invariably 'doing something', and that something may be very quiet and home-based (such as reading) or very outgoing and active (such as taking part in amateur drama). Moreover, given the way in which this question was asked, these activities can be said to be purposive in that respondents have *chosen* to put them in their activity diagram. In other words, they are potentially the means through which respondents are able to express themselves, gain enjoyment, and which contain dimensions of freedom and intrinsic satisfaction.

What, though, are the most commonly cited activities that these elderly respondents spend time doing, and which they regard as so important that it would be hard to imagine life without them? In some respects, the activities citied in Table 10.2 are the reverse of those that might have been expected from a group of older people interviewed forty

Table 10.2 Most popular activities

Activity	n	%
Reading	200	33
Gardening	177	30
Watching television	159	27
Walking	104	17
Looking after the home	100	17
Shopping	86	14
Knitting	78	13
Travel/holiday	68	11
Visiting family	60	10
Cooking	59	10

or fifty years ago. Then, reading would almost certainly have come very low down in the order of priorities. A large proportion of that earlier generation (especially the working class) would, as Ross McKibbin notes, have given up reading books after leaving school.[9] The Nuffield Foundation report in 1946 commented that it had found many cases where old people said they could not be bothered with books.[10] Books have certainly become more important now in the lives of older people; reading was the most commonly cited activity among those whom we interviewed. Many homes visited for the research had lounges cluttered with well-thumbed paperbacks, large-print books, or reference books and biographies of different kinds. This was a generation that had in a sense 'discovered books' (often in spite of rather than because of formal education), and retirement was clearly often used (eyesight permitting) to develop further the pleasures of reading.

But an even bigger change for older people has undoubtedly been the importance of television. In the 1950s, no more than one in five older people would have owned or had access to a TV. In the 1990s, virtually all older people have access to at least one set. But more than ownership, television has become of huge significance in the daily lives of retired people. In the early 1950s, even for those with a TV, viewing hours were limited, with transmission from 3 p.m. on weekdays and 5 p.m. on Sundays, and close-down at 10.30 p.m. There was also a 'toddlers' truce' between 6 and 7 p.m. to ensure that children were put to bed at a proper hour.[11] And it was sometime before television produced soap operas to rival radio's *Mrs Dale's Diary* (1948) and *The Archers* (1948). By the 1990s (despite the continued popularity of the latter), television, according to one study, had become a crucial medium for helping older people keep in touch with the world.[12]

Both reading and watching television attest to the significance of 'home' for our elderly respondents. Although it is almost certainly misleading to view home and community as alternatives, it may be argued that for our respondents the balance of interests had swung throughout their lives increasingly to the former (as some of the experiences reviewed in earlier chapters might suggest). This was a generation where homes (which for the majority in Woodford and Wolverhampton were owned) had increasingly more to offer. Homes were not only sites of a 'thousand memories', but environments in which people constructed their lives through reading, television and numerous other activities. They were also environments which people had to maintain. Our generation of older people was on the crest of the 'Do-it-yourself' wave which swept through the 1950s, the decade which launched magazines such as *Practical Householder* (1955), and *Homemaker* (1959).[13] Reflecting this, 'looking after the home' was mentioned as an important activity by 17 per cent of respondents.

But of greater significance (and more popular even than television) was gardening (mentioned by 30 per cent of those interviewed). Again, this was a generation rooted in dreams of a 'private garden'. Most of the old terrace housing which many respondents had been brought up in, or had moved from, would have had no garden to speak of. Ours is a generation (Bethnal Green excepting) which moved to homes where the garden became a major focus for activities, at first mainly for men but increasingly as part of a joint task for husband and wife (a theme again foreshadowed in the original Woodford study).

Finally, what also emerges from the list of activities in Table 10.2 is the move towards either solitary or couple-orientated activities. Again, perhaps, this is an important change from the kind of old age typical of working-class communities in the 1940s and 1950s. In Sheldon's Wolverhampton, older people shared activities on the streets or in multi-generational households. Now, they are perhaps at one and the same time less 'vigorously at home in the streets', but more focused on the home itself and the private garden (visits to 'garden centres' are now a popular activity for retired people). Most of the activities listed in Table 10.2 reflect in fact the social world of couples (or widows and widowers) rather than that of extended families (some ethnic minorities being the clear exception here). People are certainly active in retirement (as we will discuss further), but activities may be enclosed within a tightly defined social as well as geographical circle.

How much do people do?

The 600 'active' respondents between them noted a total of 2,431 activities in their diagrams, giving an average number of activities of four per person. There is some indication from our data (see Table 10.3) that the number of activities people cite decreases (albeit only slightly) with age (16 per cent of those aged seventy-five and over list between six and ten activities in their circles in comparison with 26 per cent of the under seventy-five year olds), while Woodfordians are the most active and Bethnal Greeners the least (where nearly one in ten were unable to cite any significant activity in their lives).

In each study area, women tend to be somewhat more active than the men. Not surprisingly, we also find that disability limits the numbers of activities engaged in: only thirty-nine (14 per cent) of the 272 respondents with a limiting long term illness undertake six to ten activities, compared with 103 (29 per cent) of the 355 respondents without such disability. When we control for limiting long-term illness, Woodfordians are still the most active (27 per cent of those with a disability undertake six to ten activities), but disabled Wolverhampton respondents are now less active than those in Bethnal Green (7 per cent compared with 11 per cent).

Growing old: then and now

The results from our study indicate some important continuities from the baseline studies. This seems especially true of Bethnal Green, where problems in retirement – boredom, poverty, missing contacts from work – still seem to affect a substantial minority. Some older people – to be found in all areas but more prominent in Bethnal Green – seem to have substantially withdrawn from what might be taken as a reasonable standard of daily life. In the 1950s, these people were the 'social isolates' (Townsend recorded twenty in his own study), invariably living alone,

Table 10.3 Number of activities, by area

	Wolverhampton		Bethnal Green		Woodford		Total	
	n	%	n	%	n	%	n	%
None	4	2	18	9	5	3	27	4
1–5	181	79	154	79	123	60	458	73
6–10	43	19	23	12	76	37	142	23
Totals	228	100	195	100	204	100	627	100

disconnected in vital ways from the community around them. In the 1990s, this phenomenon is still present, in ways not really dissimilar from that encountered in those early post-war years. In our late modern society, twenty-seven people in our study were unable to cite a single activity which was significant or important in their lives (eighteen of these being drawn from Bethnal Green). This group (representing 4 per cent of our total sample) were mainly white (twenty-one, or 78 per cent), predominantly very elderly (eighteen, or 67 per cent), and with the majority single and living alone (fifteen, or 56 per cent). The circumstances of two, one from Bethnal Green and one from Woodford are summarised below.

Mrs Dylan, aged eighty-three, lives alone in a ground floor flat in Bethnal Green. The flat is unkempt and rather grubby with old furniture, puzzle magazines and bric-a-brac scattered around. Mrs Dylan was interviewed at the end of February and Xmas cards from her family were still lying around the flat. She has been widowed for 10 years and has four children (two living fairly close by in Bow and Hackney). Gaunt with a head scarf which covered heavily dyed but now thinning hair, Mrs Dylan is tearful at various points of the interview as she talks about her deceased husband: 'I had a wonderful husband . . . and the Lord took him. I sit here and cry but the Lord don't bring him back. I am very, very lonely. I ain't got nobody who I could say was friendly.'

Mrs Dylan reminds us of the disconnectedness of the urban world. Her family is around her – the 'four lovely children' – but she is struggling for survival; fearful of reaching out to the networks around her:

Interviewer: Are there some days when you don't see anyone?
Mrs Dylan: Yes, very lonely.
Interviewer: Do neighbours call in?'
Mrs Dylan: No . . . I had some cakes and I thought I am not going to throw them away so I took them over and knocked on his (a neighbour's) door. He said: 'No, don't knock on my door'. I didn't want nothing. I wanted to give him something. But no, so I don't bother no more.
Interviewer: What do you do to pass the time?
Mrs Dylan: Sit here and watch the people go by. That's all . . . I sit here all day.

Mr Gibson, aged eighty-three, lives alone in a three-bedroomed terraced house in Woodford. He stays mainly in one room of the house which is itself extremely dirty and untidy. Mr Gibson was dressed in very old clothes and was wearing a dressing gown. He was interviewed in March

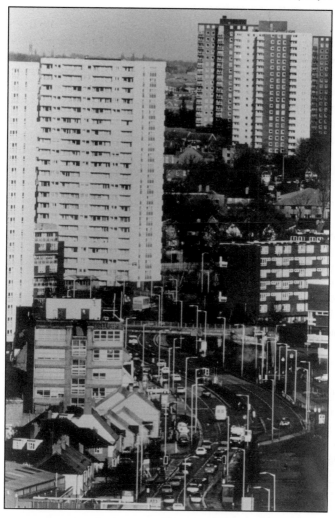

Plate 11: Heath Town, Wolverhampton, mid-1990s

Source: Picture courtesy of *Express and Star* newspaper, Wolverhampton.

but Xmas lights were still trailed around the room. His health was poor and he struggled for breath at different points in the interview. He has lived in Woodford for most of his life and in the same house since he was eight years old.

Mr Gibson identified five people in his network, all siblings. He has a widowed brother and a widowed sister living in the same street (both of whom also live alone). His brother (whose wife died fifteen years previously) provides him with support: 'He does shopping for various people. He does shopping for me. He brings me dinner every day . . . goes up the shops and gets my money at times if I can't go out.' He says of this brother: 'he does everything for me'. Mr Gibson describes himself as having always been a shy person with an 'inferiority complex'. He sees himself as cut off from relationships: 'Perhaps I am not capable of loving anybody properly, including myself. I have never been, what I would say, fond of anybody, that I know of.' Mr Gibson views the future with an emotional rawness and clarity:

> You see I am not happy. There are too many things wrong, see. I say . . . time is up. I have problems breathing, and at times quite bad . . . If you can't breathe you can't do anything. Sometimes I say to myself, 'what is the good of trying to save you, you are dying anyway'. You can't stop the dying process. I am dying. I have to accept that I am dying. I am eighty-three, see. Now all of my family have gone at about eighty or eighty-five. So I am expected to go in the next year or two. . . . I say to myself 'there is nothing you can do about it. You are dying you poor old bugger, you are dying.'
>
> And that is it. I accept it. I am dying. You see, I am not happy because I can't enjoy myself. I can't go out and enjoy myself. I am stuck here, watching TV. . . . And that is how I am today. Unhappy. Unhappy because . . . well, what is there to be happy about when you are eighty-three, in poor health, unable to enjoy yourself.

In 'deep old age' people confront the world with an emotional clarity which goes beyond simple questions of attachment or non-attachment to family. Mr Gibson had a brother who provided his main contact with the outside world; Mrs Dylan had a son and daughter who were regular visitors. But the emotional core of their lives had become detached in some way from the world around them. In inner city and suburbia, they gazed back through their lives: Mr Gibson remembered a girl in Germany who he was 'fond of' and who he had thought of marrying, Mrs Dylan a departed husband whom she dreams of endlessly. They searched for meaning in memories of the past; for some form of continuity. Their lives remind us that relationships at the end of life can be stripped to the barest of meaning: growing old as an emotional 'free fall', a constant wait for release and some kind of certainty.

Part 4

Conclusion

Chapter 11

From family groups to personal communities

Social capital and social change in old age

Introduction

The purpose of this final chapter is to present some conclusions about changes both in the family lives of our respondents, and their experience of being an older person in the three localities examined in this study. The questions here include: how have families and social networks changed over the forty to fifty years represented by our study? How different is the type of support which people receive as well as give? A further question concerns the policy dimensions related to our study, especially regarding support for families and older people within the community. As we move into a new century, issues relating to an ageing population are seen to be creating several dilemmas and concerns. To what extent do our findings add to these? Alternatively, is there a more optimistic message to be drawn from our interviews?

Older people and the family

A general finding from our research is that kinship ties have stood up well to the developments affecting urban societies over the past fifty years. Most older people are connected to family-based networks, which provide (and receive from the older person) different types of support. In respect of kinship, there is a central core to the network, which is crucial in distributing help in a variety of ways. In our study, it is clear that this core (spouses and daughters especially) is now central to the provision of emotional aid and services of different kinds. The immediate family, then, offers an important protective role to older people: reassuring in times of crisis, playing the role of confidant, and acting as the first port of call if help is needed in the home.

Our findings would, however, stress the importance of the immediate rather than the wider extended family (a point emphasised in our quantitative and qualitative data). Again, we are replicating other research by suggesting that, in general, the extended family plays a relatively limited role in the lives of older people. It does come together (as noted in Chapter 8) for birthdays, weddings and anniversaries of various kinds. But this should not be confused with more direct or active kinship roles. These, from our research, are somewhat rare: kinship relationships revolve around the immediate family (and often just one or two ties within it), rather than a large number of relationships stretching vertically through different generations and horizontally across different types of relations.

In presenting this finding, we are highlighting an important change since the baseline studies. Then (notably in Bethnal Green and Wolverhampton) older people defined their lives in the context of family groups. In Bethnal Green, a majority (54 per cent) of older people shared a dwelling with relatives. In Wolverhampton, in the 1940s, just 10 per cent of elderly people were living alone. Housing circumstances, and different fertility patterns for this cohort (see Chapter 2), contributed to a vastly different experience of old age. A major finding, in fact, from our study is that over the past fifty years, we have moved from an old age experienced largely within the context of family groups (though some ethnic minority groups have retained this form), to one where it is shaped by what Wellman has termed 'personal communities' (i.e. the world of friends, neighbours, leisure-associates and kin).[1] Close kin are still available and significant in the lives and networks of older people. They are also a major force in providing different kinds of support. We asked older people: Who is important in your life? Who provides you with support? For the majority of respondents, the answer to both questions revolved around kin.

But the way kinship is expressed is different now from how it was fifty years ago. Couples are more prominent than they were in the baseline studies; friends also have a higher profile. They are the largest single group listed in respect of intimate ties, and may play a substantial role in providing emotional support (especially for those single or widowed). This finding would appear to support Pahl and Spencer's argument about the importance of friends in contemporary society. They observe:

People grow up, parents die, children leave home, partners may come and go but some friends continue to supply support in different ways throughout the life course. With mother and father we are constrained as son or daughter. These relationships do of course change and may become increasingly friendly. However, with a true friend the relationships can grow and develop, free from the guilt and ambivalence that so often characterise family life. When things go wrong in our family or marriage we turn to a friend.[2]

Viewing older people as members of 'personal communities' bears upon an important sociological argument. The suggestion here is that in respect of social change, there is now a more 'voluntaristic' element in social relationships in old age. Fischer's research on urban social networks in the US, concluded that the concentration of population in urban settings produced an element of 'choice' in relationships so that friends played a more important role.[3] Moreover, the sociology of a 'personal community' is different from that of a family group. As was suggested in Chapter 4, the relationships of older people today are more dispersed and fragmented (if only because most older people no longer live with kin in the same household or dwelling). So there is a stronger sense now than in the baseline studies of relationships having to be 'managed' in old age. But to put this in a more positive way, the possibilities for enduring relationships in later life are probably stronger now than they were in Sheldon and Townsend's time. Geoff Mulgan expresses this point as follows:

> Contrary to the prevailing wisdom, the scope for people to make lasting relationships is greater than ever before. There may be many more divorces than in the past, but the typical successful marriage will now last forty or fifty years. Typical parents will see their children grow well into middle age. The typical friend made in adolescence will remain a potential companion for sixty or seventy years.[4]

To these general changes, however, we must also add some more specific ones which have emerged from our focus on the three particular areas. Examining the lives of people within certain localities, and comparing them with observations made at earlier points in time, has added additional insights, as well as a different dimension to our study. We now turn to consider some of the implications arising from this aspect of our work.

Changing communities and changing families

One of the objectives of our research was to say something about the experiences of older people in an urban environment. Elderly people have, we would suggest, been affected by various forms of urban development, and this is illustrated most clearly in respect of family structures and social networks. Related to this, one important finding from the research is that, in Britain today, it is misleading to talk of a single 'family life of older people'. Instead, there are a variety of family lives, each reflecting distinct types of urban change, migration histories, social class, and age relations. An argument arising from our research, therefore, is that, important though national data may be in showing general trends regarding family and household structure, there remain substantial variations when different localities are compared. This is not to say that place itself determines or shapes family life. Rather, in examining different areas one is, first, contrasting people placed in separate economic categories, and tracing the influence of these; and second, looking at the way in which communities are transformed through the process of urban change.

Of our three areas, it is clear that Bethnal Green had experienced a variety of pressures over the past fifty years, altering many aspects of the family life of older people. Certainly, as observed in Chapter 4, it is less easy now to talk about a particular kind of family life (and family structure) in Bethnal Green. The patterns range from family groups reminiscent of the 1950s to isolated men and women with residual social networks. In theoretical terms, for white respondents at least, there has been a loosening of the 'strong ties' which previously attached people to kin and neighbours. At the same time, this fragmentation has not been compensated for by material or welfare resources. In some respects, elderly people in Bethnal Green have become 'network poor'. White respondents are isolated in the sense of having insufficient strong ties on the one hand, and lacking 'weak ties' on the other. For them, the traditional network outlined by Abrams, of interdependencies between kin and neighbours, has been lost without any clear replacement.[5] Modern neighbourhoodism contains the possibility of significant commitments (among groups such as the retired) but this is largely unrealised in the Bethnal Green context, especially given the suspicion and alienation existing between white and Bengali residents (as highlighted in Chapter 5). The latter are a clear example of a group with strong ties but (in Granovetter's terms) virtually no 'weak' ties.[6] This has produced an

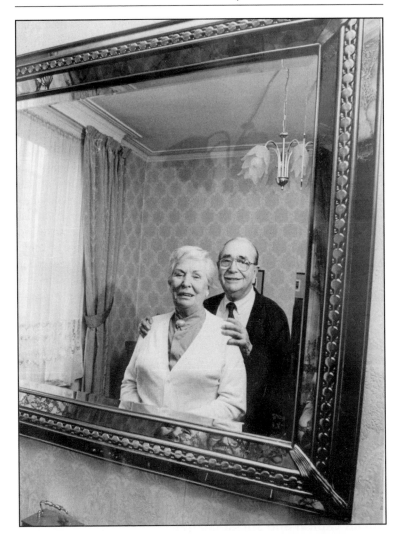

Plate 12: Pensioner couple, Bethnal Green, early 1990s

Source: Picture courtesy of Tower Hamlets Local History Library and
Archives

'encapsulated community' unable to reach out to different types of
relationships. One outcome of this is the isolation (and alienation) of
the Bengali women carers discussed in Chapter 9.

Another way of interpreting the situation of the Bethnal Green respondents concerns the issue of the social convoy. This is the group of significant others surrounding the individual. For the white, working-class residents, their social convoy seemed more open to disruption and fragmentation in respect of support. This was even more the case with the Bangladeshi older men and women, whose migration histories had introduced discontinuities in social relationships for a major part of their lives.

In the case of Wolverhampton, we suggested in Chapter 4 that there seemed to be the maintenance of a form of 'local extended family', aided by less drastic population changes than had been the case in the East End. Here, there was a sense in our findings of ties to kin and neighbours having undergone less fragmentation since Sheldon (even if they had altered in certain crucial respects). On the other hand, there was also a suggestion in our data (see some of the comments in Chapter 10) that for people losing a 'strong tie' of some kind (for example with the death of a spouse) there were few other ties to fall back upon. The issue here may be one of strong kin ties limiting the scope of relationships which can introduce people to new social ties and contacts.

Woodford respondents could be seen as examples of the 'dispersed extended family', where regular contact (weekly or more often) is maintained through the motor car and the telephone. On the one hand, this group appears as an exemplar of Rosenmayr and Kockeis' notion of 'intimacy at a distance', in some cases, pushing the logic of this attitude as far as it can possibly go.[7] On the other hand, intimacy is maintained through enduring friendships, these representing long-standing members of older people's social convoy. In this regard, the world of the Woodford elderly is at least as much friendship- as kinship-based, a pattern which was laid down in the 1950s in the move to a suburban and largely middle-class world.

Social capital and social change

The variations outlined above illustrate a more general conclusion from our study, one connected to debates in the 1990s about the changing nature of urban and community life. One suggestion, advanced for example by Robert Putnam in the US, is that since the 1960s there has been a decline in forms of civic engagement and social connectedness. Putnam sees this as amounting to a steady erosion in what he terms 'social capital', referring to: 'features of social organisation such as networks, norms, and social trust that facilitate coordination and cooperation for mutual benefit'.[8] Putnam has defined social capital according to a number of characteristics, including:

- *Community networks* which together constitute the civic community (involving institutions, associated facilities and relationships) in the voluntary, state and personal spheres, and the density of the net-working between these three spheres.
- *Civic engagement* or participation in the process of sustaining and/or using such voluntary, state and interpersonal networks.
- *Civic identity*, referring to people's sense of 'belonging' to the civic community, together with a sense of solidarity and equality with other community members.
- *Norms* governing the functioning of networks, in particular norms of *cooperation, reciprocity* (obligation to help others; confidence that others will help oneself) and *trust* (as opposed to fear) of others in the community.[9]

In Putnam's terms, the baseline studies suggested communities with high levels of social capital. Bethnal Green was viewed by Willmott and Young as somewhere which 'could have been designed expressly for aged parents, so well is it suited to their needs, providing them with company, care, and at least if they are mothers, a place of eminence in the family'. Wolverhampton provided a similar story, with Sheldon emphasising that 'to regard old people in their homes as a series of individual experiences is to miss the point of their mode of life in the community. The family is clearly the unit in the majority of instances'. In Woodford, even if the status of the old was more open to question, there was no lessening in their level of security: 'Woodford parents come to their children's door when one of them is left widowed or when both are too old or too infirm to take care of themselves any longer. From a purely physical point of view, Woodford seems to look after its old as well as in Bethnal Green.'

Taking these different examples, to what extent does our study illustrate an erosion in social capital over the post-war period? Are older people more vulnerable when localities are assessed on dimensions such as 'reciprocity' and 'support'? The stereotype would suggest this to be the case. Indeed, one argument might be that the 1950s were a 'golden age' in which to grow old given the apparent stability in family and community life. Yet, this is not a conclusion which could be drawn from our research. In the first place, to talk of a general decline in social capital is misleading. With different points of emphasis, the lives of older people in Wolverhampton and Woodford demonstrate involvement within diverse social networks, some family-focused, others with a mixture of friends, family and leisure associates. These continue to provide the mainstay of supportive needs, emotional as well as practical. And there is much to suggest reciprocity within these networks: older people are certainly providers of different kinds of help. True, the East End Mum, orchestrating an army of female kin, no longer exists. In her stead has come a more 'detached' form of intimacy, one which reflects the greater emotional investment in the couple relationship and in friendship. But intimacy – detached or otherwise – may be regarded as a valid form of social capital, one which speaks to the conditions of what Giddens and others see as a late modern age.

At the same time, we should not neglect new forms of social capital which have emerged since the 1940s and 1950s. In those decades, in a world where there were relatively few cars or telephones (especially among the old), it was meaningful to define proximity in terms of, say, five minutes walking distance (as in Sheldon's study). But near-universal access to telephones has introduced a new measure of proximity and of social capital, one highlighted in numerous ways in our interviews. Indeed, as mobile phones and e-mail become more common, there will be further substantial changes to the way social networks are defined and managed. From another vantage point, leisure activities have themselves become substantial forms of social capital, encouraging new types of engagement and participation. Retirement, albeit with some exceptions noted in Chapter 10, no longer presents the kind of stigmatisation and social withdrawal common in the 1950s. Indeed, retirement may, for some groups, represent an opportunity for expanding and developing social capital in more creative ways in comparison with previous points of the life course.

Yet it is also clear that some individuals and groups have experienced fairly major problems and, to judge from the template of the baseline studies, some of these problems are far from diminishing. It would not, for example, be reasonable to draw the conclusion now that Bethnal Green was 'designed expressly for aged parents'. On the contrary, deprivation and social exclusion of different kinds have had a marked effect on the lives of those interviewed. The family groups of Bangladeshis were reminiscent of the 1950s, but so also was the lack of space and chronic poverty. And the 'ubiquitous but camouflaged' racial prejudice of the 1950s had broken more clearly to the surface in the 1990s, undermining for some of our respondents a proper sense of security in old age. For some of the white elderly – especially those detached from the moorings of kinship – there was a sense of bewilderment about the nature of change. The language of 'insider' and 'outsider' was commonly used, but only added to the sense of exclusion. In a world of relative poverty, the wealth of the City and the new Docklands provided a sense of change over which there was no ownership. Whatever this urban world had been designed for, it was not obviously anything that had older people in mind.

All this mattered less where there were sufficient personal resources to manage and control the environment. But where resources and relationships were lacking people could feel overwhelmed by the nature of change. Some of those interviewed did seem lost and abandoned, 'waiting to die' as one respondent expressed it. Sometimes people did convey a sense of having outlived their time, missing friends and family who had gone before them. These are not 'new' feelings, and were certainly encountered in the 1950s. They do speak, however, to different forms of social exclusion in old age: at one level ideological, with the constant alarmism about the so-called burden of an ageing population; at another level attitudinal and affective, with the failure to recognise distinctive emotional needs which may surface in old age.[10] Community and personal social networks may well sustain and support (as indicated in Chapters 6 and 7), but they may also fall apart given failing health and social resources. Where this happens, the urban environment itself may provide the biggest challenge and threat to integrity and security in old age.

Developing social policy: urbanisation and community care

Our study points to the need for a new approach in respect of social policies for older people. The research has focused on issues relating to urban contexts and social networks, and, as a consequence, has highlighted new patterns of exclusion as well as inclusion among older people. We think that the debate needs to move on from generalised statements about the family life of older people (which may or may not have been true for a particular period of time). In the twenty-first century, there will almost certainly be many different family experiences, and these will raise complex issues for the development of social policy. This study (for reasons outlined in Chapter 3) has presented issues in terms of social networks, and this, for many researchers, is proving a helpful approach for thinking about relationships in old age (the work of Clare Wenger has been especially significant in this regard). From our perspective, there do seem to be a number of issues, arising from the network approach, which raise interesting policy questions.

The first set of questions concerns how we approach the issue of social support within the field of social policy. Typically, we see the family as providing the bedrock of support for older people, and this, as we noted in Chapter 2, has been a major thrust of community care policy since at least the 1980s. Our research, however, indicates some refinement may be necessary to this idea of the family as the lynchpin of what Wenger has termed the 'supportive network'.[11] In the first place, it is clear that the relationships providing help to the older person are highly focused around the immediate family. The role of spouse, daughter and son (in that order) stand out as crucial in respect of who is mobilised in the network. In one sense, this is clearly not a new finding. Indeed, it merely replicates, as we observed in Chapter 9, Townsend's original findings in Bethnal Green. But our research (reinforced by other network studies) emphasises the point that there is considerable selectivity in the way in which support is handled, and that in reality there are likely to be relatively few people actually involved. We know this because in respect of networks of 'intimates', the numbers of people are actually rather small. The average size is around nine people, but one in three of our respondents had five people or less whom they would place in a 'supportive network'. Five per cent of men had networks of just one person or less.

These characteristics raise important issues for the development of social policy in general, and community care in particular. On the positive side, most people do have someone of importance to them who is able to play a confiding, helping and supporting role in their life. But very few people have a wide choice at their disposal. Most of us are likely to list one, two or three people who are central to us, and who we feel we could go for advice on events which disturb and upset the balance of our lives. Although the relatively small number is probably true of any age (for example, people of fifty are probably no different in this respect from those of eighty), there is a difference in that eighty year olds may be sharing their problems with people of the same age with similar difficulties. This point was made in another context by Valerie Karn, in her classic study of elderly neighbours in seaside towns.[12] Moreover, the problem that has to be shared may be more critical and life-threatening than for someone of fifty. So the fact that networks are both small and focused around selected ties is important. It suggests the basis for re-framing community care for the family. The debate should move on from the level of whether families care and give support (yes they do), to questions such as: how is this support arrived at? Who is involved? What are the limits to the involvement? What specialist forms of support is the network able to provide? What is it not able to provide?

Another issue raised by our research concerns the significance of ties beyond the family. A fairly consistent finding (albeit one expressed most clearly in Woodford) is the central role of friends as a helping resource. They emerge clearly in a number of supportive roles (Chapters 8–10) notably among those without children in their networks, and especially those who are single. Again, this demonstrates the value of an approach which is cautious about viewing kinship as a unique system of support. Clearly, in most respects, kinship matters; but friends matter as well. In old age, they do not necessarily fade into the background. They do of course die, and the loss of friends can be as disturbing and distressing to an older person as the loss of kin: friends are memories of the past, are reminders of one's own mortality, are representatives of a particular social history or way of doing things. But they are also contacts who are reached out to in times of difficulty: the family gives support, it is true, but more rarely provides companionship. This was certainly echoed by many respondents in our study.

The above comments relate to policy issues of how best to support older people. But our research (reinforcing the message of the baseline studies) suggests that this can be turned on its head: that older people are themselves service providers in a number of important respects. Older people are involved in a long-term chain of support, most especially to their immediate kin (mainly children) and to friends. The data tells us a significant fact: people do not cease to be active confidants (or withdraw from other types of helping) simply because they have reached sixty-five, seventy-five or eighty-five. Staying alive in your personal community means giving it sustenance in different ways, although a natural concern with the very frail and vulnerable has tended to blind us to this important fact. However, this optimistic view needs tempering with the observation that there are those with no-one of significance left in their life (seven people reported this in our study). And of course there is a larger number than this who, although part of some of kind of network, may through illnesses such as dementia or physical disability be relatively isolated from those around them. Our study certainly confirmed the existence of such individuals, and the problems they faced in maintaining a reasonable quality of life.

Central to the issue of community care has been the delivery of effective services to people in their homes (or providing residential care if need be). In some respects there has been a major change since the baseline studies, in the provision of health and social services on a scale significantly beyond that available in the 1950s. Although an examination of these services was not part of the objectives of our work, some comments can be made arising both from the survey and the qualitative data. We can make the point that service providers do not, by and large, enter into the personal networks of older people. Indeed, as may be observed from the relevant table in Chapter 4, priests and vicars are more likely to be cited by older people as part of their networks than community carers. This, however, is hardly surprising given the type of network measure used in this study.

More disturbing, however, is that there are indications in the survey data, and certainly in the qualitative data, that for the cohort of older people we interviewed social services still have a relatively low profile in their lives. People would often say: 'I will manage for as long as possible', or 'I will make do for as long as I can'. Often this is an assertion of independence. But often, and of more concern, it reflects a fatalism or uncertainty about what is on offer. In Bethnal Green, Mrs Hart (whom we have mentioned in earlier chapters) was the main carer for her husband, who had Parkinson's disease. As a couple, in retirement, they had enjoyed going around London visiting different gardens; they were also very active churchgoers. Mrs Hart now would like a wheelchair to take her husband out occasionally, perhaps to the gardens again, but at least out of the room in which they spend most of the day and night. But where to get a wheelchair? Who has them? Doctors? Social workers? Nurses? All or none of these? Mrs Hart doesn't really know. She is tired, and trying to find out about these things simply adds to her tiredness and feelings of defeat.

To be fair, this experience could not be generalised across the areas, and this is hardly surprising given the very different state of services in the three localities. There was a much stronger sense among those in Wolverhampton of a network of services. Partly this arose from the visibility of a large metropolitan borough council;

partly, also, from what was a more substantial range of services available. Poor people by and large get poor services. This certainly seemed to be the case in Bethnal Green where, among Bangladeshi and white elderly alike, there was often a feeling of people being relatively marginal to the Welfare State that was supposed to be serving them. In Woodford, in contrast, there was a stronger sense (among a largely middle-class group) that people felt able to access services when necessary, or buy support if appropriate. Again, this suggests that just as there is no one 'family life of older people', experiences of community care are also increasingly varied.

Finally, all of these observations must be placed within the context of the starting point for this study: namely, people living in cities and experiencing old age alongside (and as part of) urban change. In this context, finding solutions to the problems of old age must also be about tackling the crisis which affects cities (a point which reaches back to the concerns of our earlier studies, notably that of Willmott and Young in *Family and Kinship in East London*). A social policy for old age must address issues about where people live and the pressures they experience in these environments. Equally, it must address how an ageing population may be seen as offering a resource which can tackle some of the problems raised by the way in which cities have developed.

Such concerns are certainly topical, highlighted both in academic work, and among commentators such as Richard Rogers. His 1995 Reith Lectures offered a major critique of the way in which cities had developed. He argued that:

> The emphasis is now on selfishness and separation rather than contact and community. In the new kinds of urban development, the activities that traditionally overlapped are organised for the purpose of maximising profit for developers or retailers. Businesses are isolated and grouped into business parks; shops are grouped in shopping centres with theatre-set 'streets' built into them; homes are grouped into residential suburbs and housing estates. Inevitably, the streets and squares of this counterfeit public domain lack the diversity, vitality and humanity of everyday city life. Worse still, the existing streets of the city are drained of commercial life and become little more than a no man's land for scurrying pedestrians or sealed private cars. People today do value convenience but they also long for genuine public life, and the crowds that pack city centres on weekends testify to this.[13]

Older people, the working-class elderly in particular, have suffered greatly from the crisis in the public environment. In our study, this was expressed in the deep sense of unease which many reported about the way in which their community had changed (see Chapter 7). People talked about their dislike of the way in which the community had 'gone down', or how they felt 'unsafe', or that people were out to get them. It is difficult to know how much this is a change from the baseline studies. After all, in the late 1940s and early 1950s, there was an undercurrent of anti-Semitism in the East End. Feelings of insecurity, then, are hardly new. What may be different now is a greater sense that people are disadvantaged by living in cities; that being old and in a city is somehow less advantageous than being old by the seaside, or in a village, or even a provincial town. So people often want to leave cities despite having lived in them for the greater part of their lives.

All of this suggests some important issues need to be tackled if people (the elderly in particular) are to be part of environments which sustain them into late old age. Cities can be disabling and threatening environments at any age. The difference is that at seventy-five or eighty-five, people may feel an even greater sense of being trapped or disadvantaged by urban decay. Rogers describes cities as acting as 'demographic magnets' through the way in which they facilitate work and foster cultural development. But we need to challenge the view that once individuals have finished with work they should be seen, or treated, as marginal to the city. In the 1950s, Willmott and Young made an eloquent case for people to be treated as a natural part of city life and to have their families around them. Whether the latter is really possible (or really desirable) seems unclear. What should be possible, however, is that people view staying in cities, into old age, as a positive choice, and not one thrust upon them because they happen to lack alternatives.

There is a further argument that might be made: if we see elderly people as service providers, as suggested earlier, then they have an active role to play as citizens in reconstructing a viable and sustainable urban future. Older people do play many roles connected with civic life (as noted in Chapter 12), but many are also estranged from this life. Perhaps the most depressing finding from this study concerned the observation that, among many working-class respondents in an inner city environment such as Bethnal Green, retirement was still associated with the beginning of old age, with feelings of being unable to occupy one's time, and (for a small number) a rejection by society. All of this suggests that, forty years on from Townsend's influential findings on this issue, much remains to be done to ensure that all older people feel able to be engaged citizens in the communities within which they live.

Conclusion

This study has tried to address some of the ways in which kinship and community is experienced by older people. Overall, our findings on this question confirm that the family has retained its influential role. It is, though, a different type of family than that of the 1950s. Indeed, an important observation from our work is that in some respects it is much less easy now to talk about the 'family life of older people'. There are many more different 'types' of older people than was the case in the 1950s, and many more different types of families (not least because we live in a multi-cultural society). But the family in some form is still central to support, even if this is often focused around a small number of network members. And other relationships certainly do matter, especially for those without children, or who are single, or who are estranged from their family. Locality also seems significant. This is not because an area necessarily produces some kinds of relations rather than others; rather, we can use locality to illustrate the important social and economic differences, and divisions, which exist among older people. Moreover, as in our study, we can show that localities do have varied histories and pathways of development, and understanding these can be important in viewing issues relating to the management and production of support. Overall, the message from this research is that family relationships continue to matter to older people, but that there are constraints: some operating through choice, others through the pressures which arise though particular life histories and particular environments. Either way, the message of diversity and variety in the family and community life of older people, is an important theme and conclusion to our investigation of family relationships and social networks.

Appendix

Personal network diagram

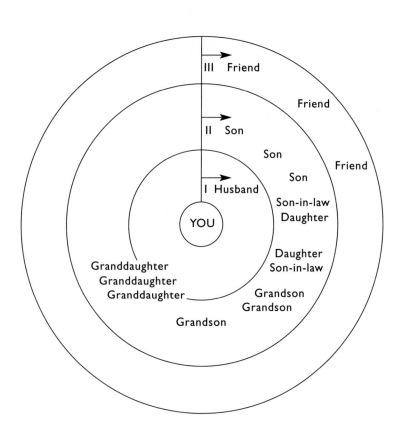

Notes

1 Growing old: other pasts; other places

1 Sheldon, *The Social Medicine of Old Age*, 1948; Townsend, *The Family Life of Old People*, 1957; Young and Willmott, *Family and Kinship in East London*, 1957; Willmott and Young, *Family and Class in a London Suburb*, 1960.
2 Frankenberg, *Communities in Britain*, 1966.
3 Laslett, 'The Significance of the Past in the Study of Ageing', 1984.
4 Willmott and Young, *Family and Class in a London Suburb*, 1960: 38.
5 Townsend, *The Family Life of Old People*, 1957: 210.
6 Goldthorpe, *Family Life in Western Societies*, 1987.
7 Cowgill and Holmes, *Aging and Modernization*, 1972.
8 Conekin, Mort and Waters, *Moments of Modernity*, 1999.
9 Crook *et al.*, *Postmodernisation*, 1992: 228.
10 Marshall, in *Sociology at the Crossroads*, 1949.
11 Lessing, *Walking in the Shade*, 1997: 5.
12 Inwood, *A History of London*, 1998: 824.
13 Rowntree, *Old People*, 1947: 32.
14 Lessing, *Walking in the Shade*: 4–5.
15 Davidoff, 'The Family in Britain', 1990.
16 Savage and Warde, *Urban Sociology*, 1993.
17 Phillips and Phillips, *Windrush: The Irresistible Rise of Multi-Racial Britain*, 1998.
18 Selvon, *The Lonely Londoners*, 1956 [1985].
19 Ibid.: 74.
20 Ibid.: 76.
21 Glass, *London's Newcomers*, 1960: 49.
22 Selvon, *The Lonely Londoners*, 1956 [1985]: 54.
23 Gardiner, *From the Bomb to the Beatles*, 1999.
24 Opie, *The 1950s Scrapbook*, 1999: 3.
25 Byatt, *The Virgin in the Garden*, 1981.
26 Young and Willmott, *Family and Kinship in East London*, 1962.
27 Riel *et al.*, *World Famous Round Here*, 1990.
28 For 'victims rather than survivors', see Williams, 'A New Age Coming', 1996: 43.
29 This literature is reviewed in Phillipson, 'The Sociology of Retirement', 1993.

30   Cumming and Henry, *Growing Old*, 1961.
31   McKibbin, *Classes and Cultures*, 1998.
32   Turner and Rennell, *When Daddy Came Home*, 1995: 224.
33   McKibbin, *Classes and Cultures*, 1998: 172–3.
34   Finch and Summerfield, 'Social Reconstruction and the Emergence of the Companionate Marriage', 1945–59', 1991.
35   Dennis *et al.*, *Coal is our Life*, 1956; Townsend, *The Family Life of Old People*, 1957.
36   Willmott and Young, *Family and Class in a London Suburb*, 1960: 132.
37   For a review of this period, see Elliott and Atkinson, *The Age of Insecurity*, 1998.
38   Rogers, 'The Making of Modern Youth', 1997.
39   Inwood, *A History of London*, 1998: 863.
40   MacInnes, *Absolute Beginners*, 1960.
41   Ibid.: 29.
42   Ibid.: 46.
43   Opie, *The 1950s Scrapbook*, 1999.
44   Moreton, 'When Saxa was Sexy', 1998: 22.
45   Willmott and Young, *Family and Class in a London Suburb*, 1960.
46   Pahl, 'Friendship', 1998: 99.
47   Elliott and Atkinson, *The Age of Insecurity*, 1998; Dunant and Porter, *The Age of Anxiety*, 1997; Fukuyama, *The Great Disruption*, 1999.
48   Beck, *The Risk Society*, 1992; Giddens, *Modernity and Self-Identity*, 1990.
49   Phillipson, *Reconstructing Old Age*, 1998.
50   Davies, *Dark Heart*, 1997; Cohn, *Yes We Have No*, 1999.
51   Fowler, *Soho Black*, 1998; Nicholson, *Bleeding London*, 1997; Nadelson, *Bloody London*, 1999; Richards, *Throwing the House out of the Window*, 1996; Abebayo, *Some Kind of Black*, 1996.
52   Sinclair, *Lights Out for the Territory*, 1997: 83.
53   Richards, *Throwing the House out of the Window*, 1996: 34.
54   Cornell, 'Does the Sun Rise Over Dagenham?', 1998: 34.
55   Berne, *A Crime in the Neighbourhood*, 1997: 9.
56   Pahl, 'Friendship', 1998: 111.
57   Lurie, *The Last Resort*, 1999.
58   Phillipson, *Reconstructing Old Age*, 1998.

2   Social networks and social support in old age

1   Wellman, *Families in Community Settings*, 1990: 195.
2   Kosberg (ed.), *Family Care of the Elderly*, 1992.
3   Townsend, *The Family Life of Old People*, 1957: 227.
4   Rosenmayr and Kockeis, 'Propositions for a Sociological Theory of Ageing and the Family', 1963.
5   Finch and Mason, *Negotiating Family Responsibilities*, 1993.
6   Jerrome, *Good Company*, 1992.
7   Willmott, *Friendships, Networks and Social Support*, 1987: 80.
8   For a comprehensive review of demographic changes see McRae (ed.), *Changing Britain*, 1999.
9   Seccombe, *Millennium of the Family*, 1993.

10 Anderson, *Family Structure in Nineteenth Century Lancashire*, 1971: 84.
11 Wall, 'Relationships Between the Generations in British Families Past and Present', 1992: 70.
12 Cited in Bourke, *Working-class Cultures in Britain 1890–1960*, 1994: 139.
13 Rosser and Harris, *The Family and Social Change*, 1965.
14 Ibid.: 302.
15 Ibid.: 285.
16 Willmott and Young, *Family and Class in a London Suburb*, 1960: 72.
17 For a review of demographic change as it affects the family see Anderson, 'What is New About the Modern Family', 1993.
18 Putnam, 'Bowling Alone', 1996: 67.
19 Barnes, 'Class and Community in a Norwegian Island Parish', 1954; Mitchell (ed.), *Social Networks in Urban Communities*, 1969.
20 Bott, *Family and Social Networks*, 1957.
21 Locality-based: Wellman and Wortley, 'Brothers' Keepers', 1989. Personal networks: Cochran *et al.*, *Extending Families*, 1990. Older adults: Antonucci and Akiyama, 'Social Networks in Adult Life', 1987.
22 Wenger, *The Supportive Network*, 1984; Wenger, 'A Comparison of Urban with Rural Networks in North Wales', 1995.
23 Bowling *et al.*, 'Life Satisfaction and Association with Social Network and Support Variables in Three Samples of Elderly People', 1991.
24 Willmott, *Friendship Networks and Social Support*: 4.
25 House and Kahn, 'Measures and Concepts of Social Support', 1985.
26 Bowling *et al.*, 'Life Satisfaction and Association with Social Networks and Support Variables', 1991: 549.
27 Pearlin, 'Social Structure and Processes of Social Support', 1985.
28 Ibid.: 44.
29 Crow and Allan, *Community Life*, 1994: 189.
30 Kahn and Antonucci, 'Convoys Over the Life Course', 1980.
31 Antonucci, 'Personal Characteristics, Social Support and Social Behaviour', 1985: 97.
32 Some examples of the impact of social networks may be found in Cochran *et al.*, *Extending Families*, 1990 and in Perri 6, *Escaping Poverty*, 1997.
33 These are summarised in Harris, 'The Family in Post-war Britain', 1994.
34 On exchange, see Wenger, *The Supportive Network*, 1984; Fischer, *To Dwell Amongst Friends*, 1982. On role relations, see Cochran *et al.*, *Extending Families*, 1990. On the subjective question, see Kahn and Antonucci, 'Convoys Over the Life Course', 1980.
35 Antonucci and Akiyama, *Social Networks in Adult Life*, 1995; Knipscheer *et al.* (eds), *Living Arrangements of Old Adults*, 1995; Lang and Cartensen, 'Close Emotional Relationships in Late Life', 1994.
36 Wenger, 'A Comparison of Urban with Rural Networks in North Wales', 1995.
37 For further details on the methodology of the study see Ogg *et al.*, *Patterns of Kinship in the Urban Environment*, 1996.
38 Office of Population Censuses and Surveys, *1995 General Household Survey*, 1996.
39 Ibid.
40 Ibid.

3 The social context of ageing: community, locality and urbanisation

1 Crow and Allan, *Community Life*, 1994.
2 Roberts *et al.*, cited in Crow and Allan, *Community Life*, 1994: xx.
3 Giddens, *Modernity and Self-Identity*, 1990.
4 Beck, *The Risk Society*, 1992.
5 Harvey, *The Condition of Post-Modernity*, 1996.
6 A theme developed by Robertson in 'Globalisation and Glocalisation', 1994.
7 Albrow, 'Travelling Beyond Local Places', 1997: 53.
8 Phillipson, 'Community Care and the Social Construction of Citizenship', 1994.
9 Stacey, 'The Myth of Community Studies', 1969.
10 *The Shorter Pepys*, 1985: 290.
11 Robb, *Working-Class Anti-Semite*, 1954: 184.
12 Porter, *London: A Social History*, 1994: 118.
13 Booth, *Life and Labour of the People of London*, 1902–3.
14 Robb, *Working-Class Anti-Semite*, 1954: 197.
15 Llewellyn-Smith, (ed.), *The New Survey of London Life and Labour*, 1934–5.
16 Vale, *Bethnal Green at War*, 1945.
17 Described in Ziegler, *London at War*, 1996: 238.
18 Glass, and Frenkel, 'How They Live at Bethnal Green', 1946: 49.
19 Cited in Frankenburg, *Communities in Britain*, 1966: 177.
20 Porter, *London: A Social History*, 1994: 342.
21 Glass, and Frenkel, 'How They Live at Bethnal Green', 1946; Robb, *Working-Class Anti-semite* 1954; Townsend, *The Family Life of Older People*, 1957; Young and Willmott, *Family and Kinship in East London*, 1957.
22 Porter, *London: A Social History*, 1994: 351.
23 Holme, *Housing and Young Families in East London*, 1985: 24.
24 Warnes, 'Migration Among Older People', 1996.
25 Frayman *et al.*, *Breadline Britain*, cited in Gordon and Forrest, *People and Places*, 1995.
26 Rix, 'Social and Demographic Change in East London', 1996.
27 Butler and Rustin, *Rising in the East*, 1996.
28 Barnsby, *Social Conditions in the Black Country, 1800–1900*, 1980.
29 For a useful review of Wolverhampton in the nineteenth century see Wallis, 'A Brief History of Victorian Wolverhampton', http://scitsc.wiv.ac.uk/-cm 1906/victorian.wton.html
30 Brennan, *Wolverhampton*, 1948.
31 Mason, *The Book of Wolverhampton*, 1979.
32 Barnsby, *Social Conditions in the Black Country*, 1800–1900, 1980: 96–8.
33 Priestley, *English Journey*, 1934: 113.
34 Brennan, *Wolverhampton*, 1948.
35 *Wolverhampton Chronicle*, August, 1950.
36 Sheldon, *The Social Medicine of Old Age*, 1948: 162.
37 *Wolverhampton Express and Star*, January 1951.
38 Medical Officer of Health, Wolverhampton, Annual Report, 1965.
39 For a superb account of childhood in a Punjabi family living in a mining village close to Wolverhampton, see Syal, *Anita and Me*, 1997.
40 Clarke, *Hope and Glory*, London, 1996: 323.

41 D. Gordon and R. Forrest, *People and Places 2*, 1995.
42 Wolverhampton Metropolitan Borough Council, Report, 1996: 9–10.
43 Louis Worth, cited in Holme, *Housing and Young Families in East London*, 1985: 13.
44 Ibid.: 13
45 Woodford Historical Society, *Woodford in the 1930s*, 1992.
46 Ibid.
47 Willmott and Young, *Family and Class in a London Suburb*, 1960: 3.
48 Ibid.: 13.

4 Household structure and social networks in later life

1 Glaser, 'The Living Arrangements of Elderly People', 7, 1997.
2 Llewellyn-Smith (ed.). *New Survey of London Life and Labour*, 1934–35.
3 Eade *et al.*, 'The Bangladeshis', 1996: 150–60.
4 Antonucci and Akiyama, 'Social Networks in Adult Life', 1987.
5 Firth, Hubert and Forge, *Families and their Relatives*, 1970.
6 For an illustration of this inter-generational theme see Attias-Donfut and Arber, *The Myth of Generational Conflict*, 2000; for an account of the role of grandparents in the family, see Thompson, 'The Role of Grandparents When Parents Part or Die', 1999.
7 A recent study reviewing the nature of friendship in modern times is Adams and Allan, *Placing Friendship in Context*, 1998.
8 Rosser and Harris, *The Family and Social Change*, 1965: 212–13.
9 Abrams, *Beyond Three-Score and Ten*, 1978.
10 Fischer, *To Dwell amongst Friends*, 1982: 175.
11 Jerrome, 'Ties that Bind', 1996.
12 Willmott, *Social Networks, Informal Care and Public Policy*, 1986: 26–7.
13 Glass and Frenkel, 'How They Live at Bethnal Green', 1946.
14 Antonucci and Akiyama, 'Social Networks in Adult Life', 1987.
15 Pearlin, 'Social Structure and Processes of Social Support', 1985.

5 Growing old in urban communities

1 Crow and Allan, *Community Life*, 1994.
2 Bulmer, *Neighbours: The Work of Philip Abrams*, 1986: 21.
3 Wenger, *The Supportive Network*, 1984: 95.
4 Rosow, *Social Integration of the Aged*, 1967.
5 Bourke, *Working-Class Cultures in Britain 1890–1960*, 1994: 156–7.
6 Roberts, *Women and Families*, 1995.
7 Ibid.: 233.
8 Gorer, *Exploring English Character*, 1955.
9 Ibid.: 52.
10 Townsend, *The Family Life of Old People*, 1957: 121.
11 Glass and Frenkel 'How They Live at Bethnal Green', 1946.
12 Robb, *Working-Class Anti-Semite*, 1954; Young and Willmott, *Family and Kinship in East London*, 1957.
13 Willmott and Young, *Family and Class in a London Suburb*, 1957: 106.

14   Young and Willmott, *Family and Kinship in East London*, 1957: 105.
15   Bulmer, *Neighbours: The Work of Philip Abrams*, 1986: 18.
16   Willmott, *Social Networks, Informal Care and Public Policy*, 1986.
17   Office of Population Censuses and Surveys, *1995 General Household Survey*, London, 1996.
18   Willmott and Young, *Family and Class in a London Suburb*, 1957: 4.
19   Roberts, *Women and Families*, 1995: 201.
20   Cohen, *Whalsay*, 1987; Cornwell, *Hard Earned Lives*, 1984.
21   Bourke, *Working-Class Cultures in Britain, 1890–1960*, 1994.
22   Klein, *Samples from English Cultures*, 1965: 13.
23   Wilkinson, *Unhealthy Societies*, 1996.
24   Taylor, Evans and Fraser, *A Tale of Two Cities*, 1996: 260.
25   Klein, *Samples from English Cultures*, 1965: 133–4.
26   Husband, 'East-End Racism 1900–1980', 1982.
27   Willmott, *The Evolution of a Community*, 1963.
28   For 'the deep, deep sleep of England', see George Orwell's *Homage to Catalonia,* 1938: 314.
29   For the late 1940s, see Glass and Frenkel, 'How They Live at Bethnal Green', 1946.
30   McKibbin, *Classes and Cultures*, 1998.
31   Ibid.

6 Social support in late life

1   Jamieson, *Intimacy*, 1998: 136.
2   Duncombe and Marsden, 'Love and Intimacy', 1993: 221–41.
3   Kunemund and Rein, 'There is More to Receiving than Needing', 1997.
4   Allan, *Kinship and Friendship*, 1996.
5   Wellman and Wortley, 'Brothers' Keepers', 1989: 299.
6   Ibid.
7   Giddens, Reith Lectures, 1999.

8 Ties that bind

1   Townsend, *The Family Life of Old People*, 1957: 83.
2   Willmott and Young, *Family and Class in a London Suburb*, 1960: 75.
3   Ibid.: 71.
4   McGlone *et al.*, 'Kinship and Friendship', 1999.
5   Ibid.
6   Qureshi, 'Responses to Dependency', 1986.

9 Family care and support in ethnic minority groups

1   Modood *et al., Ethnic Minorities in Britain*, 1997: 20.
2   Ibid.
3   Choudhury, *Roots and Tales of the Bangladeshi Settlers*, 1993.
4   Ibid.: 137.
5   Gardener, *Identity, Age and Masculinity*, 1999.

6   Ballard, *Desh Pradesh*, 1994
7   Gardener, *Narrating Location*, 1997: 9.
8   Department of Social Security, *Family Resources Survey*, 1996.
9   Silveria and Ebrahim, 'Mental Health and Health Status', 1995
10 For a description of the Life Satisfaction Index see Bowling, *Measuring Health*, 1991.
11 Department of the Environment, 1993.
12 Ahmed and Atkin, *Race and Community Care*, 1996.
13 Rudat, *Health and Lifestyles*, 1994.
14 Blakemore and Boneham, *Age, Race and Ethnicity*, 1994.
15 Cameron, *Black Older Women, Disability and Health*, 1989.
16 Selvon, *Lonely Londoners*, 1956 [1985].

10 The social world of older people

1. Townsend, *The Family Life of Old People*, 1957: 147.
2   Ibid.: 146–7.
3   Willmott and Young, *Family and Class in a London Suburb*, 1960, p.64.
4   Ibid.: 89.
5   Stearns, *Old Age in European Society*, 1977.
6   Bone *et al.*, *Retirement and Retirement Plans*, 1992.
7   Parker, *Older Workers and Retirement*, 1980: 72.
8   Glass and Frenkel, 'How They Live at Bethnal Green', 1946: 40.
9   McKibbin, *Classes and Cultures*, 1998: 499.
10 Rowntree, *Old People*, 1947: 80.
11 Gardiner, *From the Bomb to the Beatles*, 1999: 98.
12 Gauntlett and Hill, *TV Living*, 1999.
13 Opie, *The 1950s Scrapbook*, 1999.

11 From family groups to personal communities

1   Wellman, 'The Place of Kinfolk in Community Settings', 1990.
2   Pahl and Spencer, 'The Politics of Friendship', 1997
3   Fischer, *To Dwell Amongst Friends*, 1982.
4   Mulgan, *Connexity*, 1997: 153.
5   Bulmer, *Neighbours: The Work of Philip Abrams*, 1986.
6   For a valuable review of the network literature on this point see Perri, 6 *Escaping Poverty*, 1997; see also the classic essay by Granovetter, 'The Strength of Weak Ties', 1973.
7   Rosenmayr and Kockeis, 'Propositions for a Sociological Theory of Ageing and the Family', 1963.
8   Putnam, 'Bowling Alone', 1995: 67.
9   Ibid.: 7.
10 These areas are discussed in more detail in Biggs, *The Mature Imagination*, 1999 and in Phillipson, *Reconstructing Old Age*, 1998.
11 Wenger, 'The Supportive Network', 1984.
12 Karn, *Retiring to the Seaside*, 1977.
13 Rogers, *Cities for a Small Planet*, 1995: 50.

Bibliography

Abebayo, D. *Some Kind of Black*. London: Abacus, 1996.

Abrams, M. *Beyond Three Score and Ten*. London: Age Concern Research Publications, 1978.

Adams, R. and Allan, G. *Placing Friendship in Context*. Cambridge: Cambridge University Press, 1998.

Ahmed, B. and Atkin, K. *Race and Community Care*. London: Macmillan, 1996.

Albrow, M. 'Travelling Beyond Local Places: Socio-scapes in a Global City', in *Living the Global City*. London, 1997: 53.

Allan, G. *Friendship: Developing a Sociological Perspective*. Hemel Hempstead: Harvester Wheatsheaf: 1989.

—— *Kinship and Friendship in Modern Britain*. Oxford: Oxford University Press, 1996.

Allen, I. and Perkins, E. *The Future of Family Care for Older People*. London: HMSO, 1995.

Anderson, M. *Family Structure in Nineteenth Century Lancashire*. Cambridge: Cambridge University Press, 1971.

—— 'What is New About the Modern Family'. *The Family*, 31, 1993: 2–16.

Antonucci, T. 'Personal Characteristics, Social Support, and Social Behaviour', in R. Binstock and E. Shanas, *Handbook of Aging and the Social Sciences*. New York: Greenwood Press, 1985.

—— 'Convoys of Social Relations: Family and Friendships within a Life Span Context', in R. Blieszner and V. H. Bedford, *Handbook of Aging and the Family*. New York: Greenwood Press, 1995.

Antonucci, T. and Akiyama, H., 'Social Networks in Adult Life: A Preliminary Examination of the Convoy Model'. *Journal of Gerontology*, 4, 1987: 519–27.

Attias-Donfut, C. and Arber, S. *The Myth of Generational Conflict*. London: Routledge, 2000.

Ballard, R. (ed.) *Desh Pradesh: The South Asian Presence in Britain*. London: Hurst, 1994.

Barnes, J. A. 'Class and community in a Norwegian Island Parish'. *Human Relations*, 7, 1954: 39–58.

Barnsby, G. J. *Social Conditions in the Black Country, 1800–1900*. Wolverhampton: Integrated Publishing Services, 1980.

Beck, U. *The Risk Society*. Cambridge: Sage, 1992.

Berne, S. *A Crime in the Neighbourhood*. London: Penguin Books, 1997.

Biggs, S. *The Mature Imagination*. Buckingham: Open University Press, 1999.

Blakemore, K. and Boneham, M. *Age, Race and Ethnicity*. Milton Keynes: Open University Press, 1994.

Bone, M., Gregory, J., Gill, B. and Lader, D. *Retirement and Retirement Plans*. London: Office of Population Censuses and Surveys, 1992.

Booth, C. *Life and Labour of the People of London*. 3rd edn, 1902–3.

Bott, E. *Family and Social Networks*. London: Tavistock, 1957.

Bourke, J. *Working-class Cultures in Britain, 1890–1960*. London: Routledge, 1994.

Bowling, A. *Measuring Health*. Buckingham: Open University Press, 1997.

Bowling, A., Farquhar, M. and Browne, P. 'Life Satisfaction and Association with Social Network and Support Variables in Three Samples of Elderly People'. *International Journal of Geriatric Psychiatry*, 6, 1991: 549–66.

Brennan, T. *Wolverhampton: Social and Industrial Survey 1945–1946*. London: Dennis and Dobson, 1948.

Bulmer, M. *Neighbours: The Work of Philip Abrams*. Cambridge: Cambridge University Press, 1986.

—— *The Social Basis of Community Care*. London, Allen and Unwin, 1987.

Butler, T. and Rustin, M. *Rising in the East: The Regeneration of East London*. London: Lawrence and Wishart, 1996.

Byatt, A. S. *The Virgin in the Garden*. London: Penguin Books, 1981.

Cameron, E. *Black Older Women, Disability and Health*. London: Routledge, 1989.

Choudhury, Y. *Roots and Tales of the Bangladeshi Settlers*. Birmingham: Sylhet Social History Group, 1993.

Clarke, P. *Hope and Glory: Britain 1900–1990*. London: Allen Lane, 1996.

Cochran, M., Larner, M., Riley, D., Gunnarsson, S. and Henderson, C. *Extending Families*. Cambridge: Cambridge University Press, 1990.

Cohen, A. *Whalsay: Symbol, Segment and Boundary in a Shetland Island Community*. Manchester: Manchester University Press, 1987.

Cohn, N. *Yes We Have No: Adventures in Other England*. London: Secker and Warburg, 1999.

Conekin, B., Mort, F. and Waters, C. *Moments of Modernity: Reconstructing Modernity*. London: Rivers Oram Press, 1999.

Cornell, D. 'Does the Sun Rise Over Dagenham?', in *Does the Sun Rise Over Dagenham: New Writing from London*, London: Fourth Estate, 1998.

Cornwell, J. *Hard Earned Lives*. London: Tavistock, 1984.

Cowgill, D. O. and Holmes, D. (eds), *Ageing and Modernization*. New York: Appleton-Century-Crofts, 1972.

Crook, S., Pakulski, J. and Waters, M. *Postmodernization*. London: Sage, 1992.

Crow, G. and Allan, G. *Community Life: An Introduction to Local Social Relations*. Hemel Hempstead: Harvester Wheatsheaf, 1994.

Cumming, E. and Henry, W. E. *Growing Old, The Process of Disengagement*. New York: Basic Books, 1961.

Davidoff, L. 'The Family in Britain', in F. M. Thompson, *People and their Environment*, vol.2. The Cambridge Social History of Britain. Cambridge: Cambridge University Press, 1990: 71–129.

Davies, N. *Dark Heart: The Shocking Truth About Hidden Britain*. London: Vintage, 1998.

Dennis, N., Henriques, F. and Slaughter, C. *Coal is Our Life*. London: Tavistock, 1956.

Department of the Environment *English Housing Condition Survey 1991*. London: HMSO, 1993.

Dunant, S. and Porter, R (eds), *The Age of Anxiety*. London: Virago Press, 1997.

Duncombe, J. and Marsden, D. 'Love and Intimacy: The Gender Division of Emotion and "Emotion Work"'. *Sociology*, 27, 1993: 221–41.

Eade, J., Vamplew, T. and Peach, C. 'The Bangladeshis: The Encapsulated Community', in *Ethnicity in the 1991 Census*: vol. 2: *The Ethnic Minority Populations of Britain*. London: HMSO, 1996.

Elliott, L. and Atkinson, D. *The Age of Insecurity*. London: Verso, 1998.

Finch, J. *Family Obligations and Social Change*. Cambridge: Polity, 1989.

—— 'Responsibilities, Obligations and Commitments', in I. Allen and E. Perkins (eds), *The Future of Family Care for Older People*. London: HMSO, 1995: 51–64.

Finch, J. and Mason, J. *Negotiating Family Responsibilities*. London: Routledge, 1993.

Finch, J. and Summerfield, P. 'Social Reconstruction and the Emergence of the Companionate Marriage', in D. Clark (ed.), *Marriage, Domestic Life and Social Change*. London: Routledge, 1991: 7–32.

Firth, R., Hubert, J. and Forge, A. *Families and their Relatives*. London: Routledge, 1970.

Fischer, C. S. *To Dwell Amongst Friends*. Chicago: University of Chicago Press, 1982.

Fowler, C. *Soho Black*. London: Warner, 1998.

Frankenburg, R. *Communities in Britain*. London: Penguin, 1966.

Frayman, H., Mack, J., Lansley, S., Gordon, D. and Hills, J. *Breadline Britain – 1990s: The Findings of the Television Series*. London: Domino Films and London Weekend Television, 1991.

Fukuyama, F. *The Great Disruption: Human Nature and the Reconstitution of the Social Order*. London: Profile Books, 1999.

Gardener, K. *Narrating Location: Space, Age and Gender among Bengali Elders in East London*. Mimeo, 1997.

—— 'Identity, Age and Masculinity among Bengali Elders in East London', in A. Kershen (ed.), *A Question of Identity*. London: Ashgate, 1999.

Gardiner, J. *From the Bomb to the Beatles*. London: Collins and Brown, 1999.

Gauntlett, D. and Hill, A. *TV Living-Television, Culture and Everyday Life*. London: Routledge, 1999.

Giddens, A. *Modernity and Self-Identity*. Cambridge: Polity Press, 1990.

—— 1999 Reith Lectures, Lecture No. 4.
http://news.bbc.co.uk/hi/english/static/events/reik_99/week4/htm.

Glaser, R. 'The Living Arrangements of Elderly People'. *Reviews in Clinical Gerontology*. 7, 1997: 63–72.

Glass, R. *London's Newcomers*. Cambridge, Mass.: Harvard University Press, 1961.

Glass, R. and Frenkel, M. 'How They Live At Bethnal Green', in *Britain Between East and West*. London: Contact Books, 1946.

Goldthorpe, J. E. *Family Life in Western Societies*. Cambridge: Cambridge University Press, 1987.

Gordon, C. *The Myth of Family Care? The Elderly in the Early 1930s*. London: The Welfare State Programme, London School of Economics, 1988.

Gordon, D. and Forrest, R. *People and Places 2: Social and Economic Distinctions in England*. Bristol: School for Advanced Urban Studies, 1995.

Gorer, G. *Exploring English Character*. London: Cresset Press, 1955.

Granovetter, M. 'The Strength of Weak Ties'. *American Journal of Sociology*, 78, 1973: 1360–80.

Grieco, M. 'Transported Lives: Urban Social Networks and Labour Circulation', in A. Rogers, and A. Vertovec (eds), *The Urban Context*. Oxford, Berg, 1995.

Harvey, D. *The Condition of Postmodernity*. Oxford: Oxford University Press, 1996.

Holme, A. *Housing and Young Families in East London*. London: Routledge, 1985.

Hough, M. *Anxieties about crime: findings from the 1994 British Crime Survey Research Study 147*. Home Office Research and Statistics Department. London: Home Office, 1995.

House, J. and Kahn, R. 'Measures and Concepts of Social Support', in S. Cohen and L. Syme (eds), *Social Support and Health*. New York: Academic Press, 1985.

Husband, C. 'East End Racism 1900–1980'. *London Journal*, 8, 1982: 3–26.

Inwood, S. *A History of London*. London: Macmillan, 1998.

Jamieson, L. *Intimacy*. Cambridge: Polity, 1998.

Jerrome, D. *Good Company: an Anthropological Study of Older People in Groups*. Edinburgh: Edinburgh University Press, 1992.

Jerrome, D. 'Ties that Bind', in A. Walker (ed.), *The New Generational Contract: Intergenerational Relations, Old Age and Welfare*. London: UCL Press, 1996.

Kahn, R. and Antonucci, T. 'Convoys over the Life Course: Attachment, Roles and Social Support', in P. B. Baltes and O. Brim, *Life-Span Development and Behaviour*, vol. 3. New York: Academic Press, 1980.

Karn, V. *Retiring to the Seaside*. London: RKP, 1977.

Klein, J. *Samples from English Cultures*. London: RKP, 1965.

Knipscheer, K. and Antonucci, T. (eds), *Social Network Research: Substantive Issues and Methodological Questions*. Amsterdam: Swets and Zeitlinger, 1990.

Knipscheer, K., Van de Jong Gieveld, J., Tilburg, T. G. and Dykstra, P. A. (eds), *Living Arrangements and Social Networks of Older Adults*. Amsterdam: VU University Press, 1995.

Kosberg, J. (ed.) *Family Care of the Elderly*. London: Sage Books, 1992.

Kunemund H. and Rein, M. 'There is More to Receiving than Needing: Theoretical Arguments and Empirical Explorations on Crowding In and Crowding Out'. *Mimeo*, 1997.

Lang, F. and Cartensen, L. 'Close Emotional Relationships in Later Life: Further Support for Proactive Aging in the Social Domain'. *Psychology and Aging*, 9, 1994: 315–24.

Laslett, P. 'The Significance of the Past in the Study of Ageing'. *Ageing and Society*, 4, 1995: 379–89.

Latham, R. (ed.) *The Shorter Pepys*. London: Bell and Hyman, 1985.

Lessing, D. *Walking in the Shade*. London: Flamingo, 1997.

Llewellyn-Smith, H. (ed.) *The New Survey of London Life and Labour*, London: P. S. King, 1934–5.

Lurie, A. *The Last Resort*. London: Vintage, 1999.

McCallister, L. and Fischer, C. 'A Procedure for Surveying Personal Networks'. *Sociological Methods and Research*, 7, 1978: 131–47.

McGlone, F. Park, A. and Roberts, C. 'Kinship and Friendship: Attitudes and Behaviour in Britain, 1986–1995', in S. McRae (ed.), *Changing Britain: Families and Households in the 1990s*. Oxford: Oxford University Press, 1999.

Macinnes, C. *Absolute Beginners*. London: Macgibbon and Kee, 1960.

McKibbin, R. *Classes and Cultures: England 1918–1951*. Oxford: Oxford University Press, 1998.

McRae, S. (ed.) *Changing Britain: Families and Households in the 1990s*. Oxford: Oxford University Press, 1999.

Marshall, T. H. *Sociology at the Crossroads*. London: Heinemann, 1963.

Mason, F. *The Book of Wolverhampton*. Buckingham: Barracuda, 1979.

Mitchell, J. C. (ed.) *Social Networks in Urban Communities*. Manchester: Manchester University Press, 1969.

Modood, T. *et al. Ethnic Minorities in Britain*. London: Policy Studies Institute, 1997.

Moreton, C. 'When Saxa was Sexy'. *Independent on Sunday*, 1 November, 1998: 22.

Mulgan, G. *Connexity: How to Live in a Connected World*. London: Chatto and Windus, 1997.

Nadelson, R. *Bloody London*. London: Faber and Faber, 1999.

Obelkevich, J. and Catterall, P. (eds) *Understanding Post-War British Society*. London: Routledge, 1994.

Office of Population Censuses and Surveys, *General Household Survey*. London: Stationery Office, 1995 and 1996.

Ogg, J., Bernard, M., Phillips, J. and Phillipson, C. *Patterns of Kinship in the Urban Environment: Methodology of the 1995 Survey Phase*. Centre for Social Gerontology, Keele: University of Keele, 1996.

Opie, R. *The 1950s Scrapbook*. London: New Cavendish, 1999.

Pacione, M. *Britain's Cities: Geographies of Division in Urban Britain*. London: Routledge, 1996.

Pahl, R. 'Friendship: The Social Glue of Contemporary Society', in J. Franklin, *The Politics of Risk Society*. Cambridge: Polity Press, 1998.

Pahl, R. and Spencer, L. 'The Politics of Friendship. *Renewal*, 5, 3/4: 100–7, 1997.

Parker, S. *Older Workers and Retirement*. London: Office of Population Censuses and Surveys: Social Survey Division, 1980.

Pearlin, L. 'Social Structure and Processes of Social Support', in S. Cohen and L. Syme (eds), *Social Support and Health*. New York: Academic Press, 1985.

Perri, 6. *Escaping Poverty: From Safety Nets to Networks of Opportunity*. London: Demos, 1997.

Phillips, M. and Phillips, T. *Windrush: The Irresistable Rise of Multi-Racial Britain*. London: Harper Collins, 1998.

Phillipson, C. 'The Sociology of Retirement', in J. Bond, P. Coleman and S. Peace, *Ageing in Society*. London: Sage Books, 1993.

—— 'Community Care and the Social Construction of Citizenship'. *Journal of Social Work Practice*, 8, 1994: 103–12.

—— *Reconstructing Old Age: New Agendas in Social Theory and Social Policy*. London: Sage, 1998.

Phillipson, C., Bernard, M., and Strang, P. *Dependency and Interdependency in Old Age*. London: Croom Helm, 1986.

Phillipson, C., Bernard, M., Phillips, J. and Ogg, J. 'The Family and Community Life of Older People: Household Composition and Social Networks in Three Urban Areas'. *Ageing and Society*, 18, 1998: 259–90.

Political and Economic Planning, *Population Policy in Great Britain*. London: PEP, 1948.

Porter, R. *London: A Social History*. London: Hamish Hamilton, 1994.

Priestley, J. W. B. *English Journey*. London: Heinemann in association with Victor Gollancz, 1934.

Putnam, R. 'Bowling Alone: America's Declining Social Capital', *Journal of Democracy*, 6, 1995: 67.

Qureshi, H. and Walker, A. *The Caring Relationship*. London: Macmillan, 1989.

Richards, B. *Throwing the House out of the Window*. London: Headline, 1996.

Riel, R. V., Fowler, O and Malkin, H., *World Famous Round Here: The Photographs of Jack Hulme*. Castleford: Yorkshire Art Circus in association with Wakefield Metropolitan District Council, 1990.

Rix, V. 'Social and Demographic Change in East London', in T. Butler and M. Rustin (eds), *Rising in the East: The Regeneration of East London*. London: Lawrence and Wishart, 1996.

Robb, J. *Working-Class Anti-Semite*. London: Tavistock, 1954.

Roberts, E. *Women and Families: An Oral History 1940–1970*. Oxford: Blackwell, 1995.

Robertson, R. 'Globalisation and Glocalisation'. *Journal of International Communication*, 1, 1994: 33–52.

Roche, J. and Tucker, S. (eds), *Youth in Society*. London: Sage, 1997.

Rogers, R. *Cities for a Small Planet*. London: Faber, 1995.

Rosenmayr L. and Kockeis, E. 'Propositions for a Sociological Theory of Ageing and the Family'. *International Social Science Journal*, 15, 1963: 410–26.

Rosow, I. *Social Integration of the Aged*. New York: The Free Press, 1967.

Rosser, C. and Harris, C. C. *The Family and Social Change*. London: Routledge, 1965.

Rowntree, B. S. *Old People: Report of a Survey Committee on the Problems of Ageing and the Care of Old People*. Published for the Trustees of the Nuffield Foundation, Oxford: Oxford University Press, 1947.

Royal Commission on Population (1945–9) Report. London: HMSO, 1949.

Rudat, K. *Health and Lifestyles: Black and Minority Ethnic Groups in England*. London: Health Education Authority, 1994.

Savage, M. and Warde, A. *Urban Sociology, Capitalism and Modernity*. London: Macmillan, 1993.

Seccombe, W. *Millennium of the Family: Feudalism to Capitalism in Northwest Europe*. London: Verso Books, 1993.

Selvon, S. *The Lonely Londoners*. London: Longman, 1995.

Sheldon, S. H. *The Social Medicine of Old Age*. Oxford: Oxford University Press, 1948.

Silveria, E. and Ebrahim, S. 'Mental Health and Health Status of Elderly Bengalis and Somalis in London'. *Age and Ageing* 24: 474–80.

Sinclair, I. *Lights Out for the Territory*. London: Granta, 1997.

Sonderen, E. van, Ormel, B., Brilman, E. and van den Heuvell, C. 'Personal Network Delineation: A Comparison of the Exchange, Affective and Role-Relation Approaches', in K. Knipscheer and T. Antonucci (eds), *Social Network Research: Substantive Issues and Methodological Questions*. Amsterdam: Swets and Zeitlinger, 1990.

Stacey, M. 'The Myth of Community Studies'. *British Journal of Sociology*, 20, 1969: 134–47.

Stearns, P. *Old Age in European Society*. London: Croom Helm, 1977.

Syal, M. *Anita and Me*. London: Flamingo, 1997.

Taylor, I., Evans, K. and Fraser, P. *A Tale of Two Cities: A Study in Manchester and Sheffield.* London: Routledge, 1996.

Thompson, P 'The Role of Grandparents When Parents Part or Die'. *Ageing and Society,* 19, 1999: 471–503.

Townsend, P. *The Family Life of Old People.* London: Routledge and Kegan Paul, 1957.

Turner, B. and Rennell, T., *When Daddy Came Home: How Family Life Changed Forever in 1945.* London: Hutchinson, 1995.

Vale, G. *Bethnal Green at War.* London: Council of the Metropolitan Borough of Bethnal Green, 1945.

van Groenou, M. B. and van Tilburg, T. 'Network Analysis', in J. Birren (ed.), *Encyclopedia of Gerontology.* New York: Academic Press, 1996: 197–210.

Wall, R. 'Relationships Between the Generations in British Families Past and Present', in C. Marsh, and S. Arber, *Families and Households.* London: Macmillan, 1992.

—— 'Elderly Persons and Members of Their Households in England and Wales from Preindustrial Times to the Present', in D. Kertzer and P. Laslett (eds), *Ageing in the Past.* Berkeley: University of California Press, 1994.

Warnes, A. 'Migration Among Older People'. *Reviews in Clinical Gerontology,* 6, 1996: 101–44.

Wellman, B. 'The Place of Kinfolk in Personal Community Settings', in B. Wellman (ed.), *Families in Community Settings: Interdisciplinary Settings.* New York: Haworth Press, 1990.

—— *Families in Community Settings: Interdisciplinary Settings.* New York: Haworth, 1990.

—— 'The Place of Kinfolk in Community Settings'. *Marriage and Family Review,* 18, 1990: 195–228.

Wellman, B. and Wortley, S. 'Brothers' Keepers: Situating Kinship Relations in Broader Networks of Social Support'. *Sociological Perspectives,* 32, 1989: 273–306.

Wenger, G. C. *The Supportive Network.* London: George Allen and Unwin, 1984.

—— *Help in Old Age.* Liverpool: Liverpool University Press, 1992.

—— 'A Comparison of Urban with Rural Networks in North Wales'. *Ageing and Society,* 15, 1995: 59–82.

—— 'Social Networks and Gerontology'. *Reviews in Clinical Gerontology,* 6, 1996: 285–93.

Widgery, D. *Some Lives! A GP's East End.* London: Sinclair-Stevenson, 1991.

Wilkinson, R. *Unhealthy Societies.* London: Routledge, 1996.

Williams, V. 'A New Age Coming'. *Guardian Weekend,* September 1996: 43.

Willmott, P. *The Evolution of a Community.* London: Routledge, 1963.

—— *Social Networks, Informal Care and Public Policy.* London: Policy

Studies Institute, 1986.

—— *Friendships, Networks and Social Support*. London: Policy Studies Institute, 1987.

Willmott, P. and Young, M. *Family and Class in a London Suburb*. London: Routledge and Kegan Paul, 1957.

Woodford Historical Society, *Woodford in the 1930s*. Woodford, 1992.

Young, M. and Willmott, P. *Family and Kinship in East London*. London: Routledge and Kegan Paul, 1957.

Ziegler, P. *London at War*. London: Mandarin, 1996.

Index